Reimbur ts

PUBLICATIONS • CONSU RE

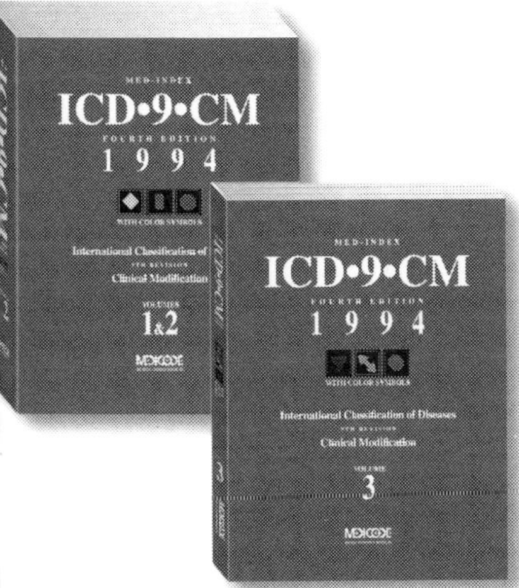

1994 ICD•9, FOURTH EDITION, VOLUMES 1, 2 & 3

NEW COLOR SYMBOLS FOR INSTANT COMPREHENSION

We're confident when we say our *1994 ICD•9* is the best on the market. Under contract with the National Center for Health Statistics, Med-Index produced the addendum and update material to the *1993 ICD•9, Volumes 1 & 2*. The Health Care Financing Administration has chosen us to produce the official *1994 ICD•9, Volume 3* for the second consecutive year. These contracts mean we can provide you with accurate, high quality ICD•9s.

Med-Index also offers new *1994 ICD•9s* with color symbols, developed to improve coding accuracy. Existing color-coded ICD•9s require memorization of more than ten colors; our three color icons simplify the coding process and are easy to remember. Our ICD•9s include:

- Attachable Quick Tabs™ and color-coded tabs for easy access to the sections you use most often.
- Definitions for ICD•9 conventions and punctuation.
- Clinical scenarios explaining common coding problems.
- Easy-to-read type printed on high quality paper.

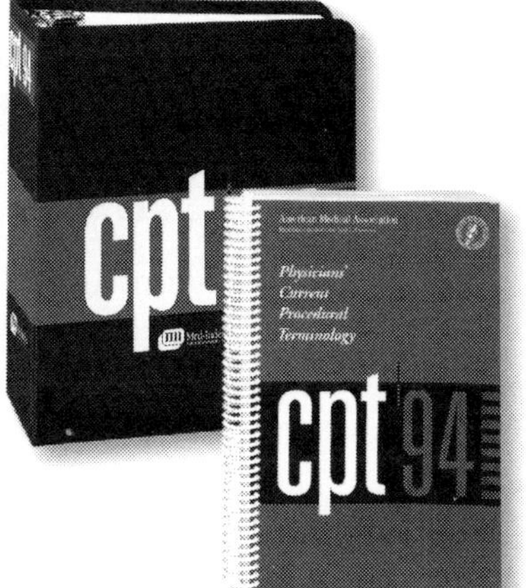

1994 CPT

CPT INCLUDES NEW CLINICAL EXAMPLES SUPPLEMENT

To help you keep up with annual changes in CPT codes, Med-Index offers *1994 CPT*, the definitive reference for procedural coding. The *Clinical Examples Supplement* illustrates scenarios for each Evaluation and Management code.

Med-Index 3-Ring Binder

- Protects contents with a durable, hard cover.
- Tabs offer easy reference to CPT sections.

Med-Index Speedy Spiral™ with Quick Tabs™

- High quality wire-o spine lies flat when open.
- Provides Quick Tabs™ with every volume. These stick-on tabs — visible from both directions — enable you to mark all sections or just the ones you frequently use.

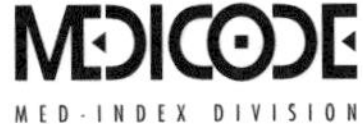

Available From Your Medical Bookstore Or Call 1-800-999-4600.
For Information On Consulting, Databases, Training And Software, Call 1-800-999-4614.

CODING ILLUSTRATED

The Eyeball

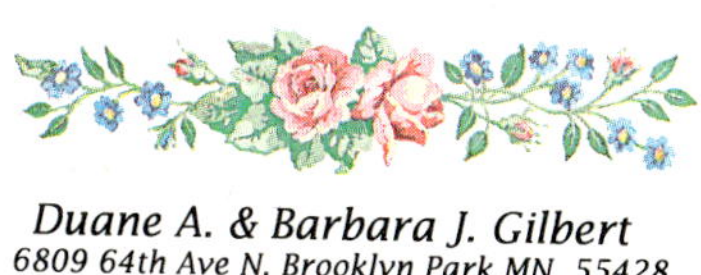

Duane A. & Barbara J. Gilbert
6809 64th Ave N, Brooklyn Park MN 55428

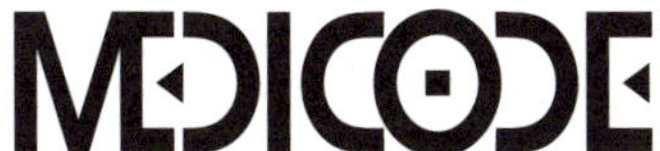

First printing December 1993

ISBN 1-56337-061-1

MEDICODE

Med-Index Publications
5225 Wiley Post Way, Suite 500
Salt Lake City, UT 84116-2889

Med-Index Publications

Series Editor	Jerry G. Seare, MD
Technical Editor	Howard A. Katzman, MD
Editorial Director	Susan P. Seare
Associate Editor	Lynn Speirs
Series Coordinator	Sheri Poe Bernard
Art Director	Paul Driscoll
Illustrators	David Hall Mike Overton Amy Shier
Technical Support	Diane McEntire Marcella Scouthern Erin Head Darby Long, RN Karen Hancock
Data Management	Rodney R. Fredette Michael W. Gifford

Special thanks to the coding experts and medical professionals at Medicode, Inc. Their knowledge, whether tapped to resolve individual reimbursement issues specific to this volume, or accessed through Medicode databases, proved an invaluable resource for the compilation of this book.

Medicode Notice

This *Coding Illustrated* volume is designed to be an accurate and authoritative source of information about coding and reimbursement issues affecting the eyeball. Every effort has been made to verify accuracy and all information is believed reliable at the time of publication. Absolute accuracy cannot be guaranteed, however. This publication is made available with the understanding that the publisher is not engaged in rendering legal or other services that require a professional license.

American Medical Association Notice

CPT is a listing of descriptive terms and five-digit numeric identifying codes and modifiers for reporting medical services performed by physicians. This presentation includes only CPT descriptive terms, numeric identifying codes and modifiers for reporting medical services and procedures that were selected by Medicode, for inclusion in this publication.

The most current CPT is available from the American Medical Association.

No fee schedules, basic unit values, relative value guides, conversion factors or scales or components thereof are included in CPT. The AMA is not recommending that any specific relative values, fees, fee schedules or related listings be attached to CPT. Any relative value scales or related listing assigned to the CPT codes are not those of the AMA and the AMA is not recommending use of these relative values.

Medicode has selected certain CPT codes and service/procedure descriptions and assigned them to various specialty groups. The listing of a CPT service or procedure description and its code number in this publication does not restrict its use to a particular specialty group. Any procedure or service in this publication may be used to designate the services rendered by any qualified physician.

The AMA assumes no responsibility for the consequences attributable to or related to any use or interpretation of any information or views contained in or not contained in the publication.

Foreword

A publication of the scope of *Coding Illustrated* requires the concerted efforts of many clinical and editorial specialists. Med-Index Publications is in the unique position of belonging to a parent company, Medicode, Inc., that serves both healthcare providers and payers. From this middle ground position has grown the expertise and insight to evaluate the thousands of coding rules and decisions necessary to present a view acceptable to both sides of reimbursement.

This ideal reference correlates CPT codes to ICD-9 and HCPCS Level II codes while providing valuable data on payer policies for follow-up days, surgical assists, prior approval, anesthesia codes, and codes that should not be billed together. Illustrations serve to educate coders about the nature of the procedures and offer clues to some of the involved nomenclature. Each installment in the series is a shortcut to the accumulated knowledge and proficiency ordinarily earned through years of coding medical procedures.

We plan to publish as many as 36 volumes of *Coding Illustrated* over the next three years. This is an ambitious goal given the research, time, and experience required of each volume. In addition to *The Eyeball,* our early volumes of *Coding Illustrated* will cover the nonpregnant uterus, tubes, and ovaries; the lower face; the ear, and the peripheral vascular system. Watch our catalog or call our sales office to check publication schedules of volumes of particular interest to your practice.

Jerry G. Seare, MD
Medical Director, Medicode, Inc.
Series Editor, *Coding Illustrated*

Introduction

Without question, a medical coder's responsibilities are enormous. Every year, changes to the *International Classification of Diseases, Ninth Revision, Clinical Modification* (ICD·9) and the American Medical Association's *Physicians' Current Procedural Terminology* (CPT) constitute a rewrite of diagnostic and procedural coding rules. At the same time, the coder is expected to know the acceptable parameters of care for each medical procedure: Is this visit part of the surgical package, or is it separately billable? Is an assistant-at-surgery generally allowed for this procedure? Finding the answers takes time and ingenuity.

From single-physician offices to multispecialty clinics and hospitals, an increasing number of office and reimbursement managers are searching for solutions to make coding easier, more accurate, and less time-consuming. Med-Index Publications has developed the *Coding Illustrated* series to be the solution to these coding problems.

Coding Illustrated allows coders to reference, in a single volume, the most essential information pertaining to a specific organ system or anatomic structure. This approach eliminates any turf wars associated with sorting codes into specialties. Clinical experts have combed through CPT to determine the system/structure-specific code set for each volume. Laboratory and radiology codes specific to that system/structure are included in the appendixes.

Because the AMA has restricted the number of CPT codes allowed in a single *Coding Illustrated* volume, a specific organ system sometimes requires more than a single book. *The Eyeball*, for instance, will be followed by a companion books *Eye Muscles and Adnexa* and *Vision*.

Coding Illustrated brings to light the nuances and complexities of procedural coding with simple illustrations, descriptions, and data relating to a specific code (e.g., postoperative follow-up days and codes that should not be billed with the code being referenced). This information can be helpful in determining what many payers consider usual and customary for a given procedure. Conversely, this data can help payers determine whether a claim falls within customary parameters. Furthermore, with the growing national emphasis on diagnostic coding, *Coding Illustrated* lists the ICD·9 codes most commonly associated with the procedure as well as billable HCPCS Level II codes for outpatient services.

CPT Code or Range

CPT Description

This verbatim description comes from the American Medical Association's *1993 Physicians' Current Procedural Teminology.*

Explanation

The procedure is described here in easy-to-understand terms.

Comments

Coding tips, insights, and references to other related codes appear in this field.

ICD•9 Procedural Codes

The most commonly associated ICD•9 Volume 3 procedural codes and their descriptions are listed here. They are taken directly from the *International Classification of Diseases, Ninth Revision, Clinical Modification (ICD•9).*

Follow-up Days
Number of follow-up days included in the global service.

Assist at Surgery
Can an assistant surgeon be billed with this procedure?

Prior Approval
Identifies an invasive, elective procedure that has been frequently or is potentially overused.

Anesthesia Code(s)
An anesthesia code, if applicable to the procedure, appears here.

Should Not Be Billed
These codes are considered incidental to or an integral part of the code described on the page and should not be billed with that code.

2

Format

The basic format of *Coding Illustrated* presents the descriptions, billing data, commentary, related ICD·9 and HCPCS Level II codes, and illustrations for each CPT code (or family of related codes) on a two-page spread. For quick identification, the code or range of codes appears in the upper left- and right-hand corners of the spread. The complete code description from CPT is placed beneath the code on the left-hand page, followed by a detailed explanation of the procedure in understandable language.

CPT CODE OR RANGE

Commonly Associated ICD•9 Diagnostic Codes

The most commonly associated ICD•9 volumes 1 and 2 diagnostic codes and their descriptions are listed here. They are taken directly from the *International Classification of Diseases, Ninth Revision, Clinical Modification (ICD•9).*

Applicable HCPCS Level II Codes

The HCPCS Level II codes commonly billed with the procedure appear here with their descriptions. Remember, HCPCS Level II codes cannot be billed for inpatient procedures.

The illustration depicts one common method of performing this procedure.

PROCEDURE NAME

3

CPT Codes and Descriptions

CPT is a standardized system of five-digit codes and descriptive terms used to report the medical services and procedures performed by physicians. It is the most widely accepted procedural coding system in the United States. In fact, all Medicare and state Medicaid carriers are required by law to use these codes for the payment of health insurance claims, and most commercial insurance payers recognize only CPT.

Indented Procedures

Understanding the indented format of CPT is critical to the proper use of CPT and *Coding Illustrated.* At first glance, some CPT code descriptions appear to be incomplete and subordinate to a code listed previously, when in fact, each description has been developed to stand alone. This format is employed to conserve space on the printed page. CPT codes that share a common procedure are grouped together, and the common procedure is fully listed only with the first code. The codes that follow are indented to indicate that a portion of their descriptions is found in a previous code.

For example:

66700 Ciliary body destruction; diathermy
66710   cyclophotocoagulation

The common portion of these two codes precedes the semicolon (;) in the full code description of code 66700. The complete description of code 66710 is:

66710 Ciliary body destruction; cyclophotocoagulation

When the data for indented procedures (e.g., follow-up days and anesthesia code) is similar to the code with the full description, *Coding Illustrated* lists them on the same page as a range of codes. When the data varies significantly, the codes are presented on separate pages. *Coding Illustrated* lists the full description for indented procedures when they are separated from the code with the full description. In some cases, two indented codes are listed on the same page as a range of codes. When this occurs, *Coding Illustrated* lists the full description with the first code and indents the second code to indicate a portion of its description is found in the previous code.

Unlisted CPT Codes

CPT provides a method for reporting procedures that have not been assigned a code. Use 66999 *Unlisted procedure, anterior segment of eye* or 67299 *Unlisted procedure, posterior segment* for unlisted procedures of the eyeball. Be aware that insurance payers review unlisted procedure codes manually, increasing processing time and the need for documentation. However, in the case of eye surgery, there is found in CPT some middle ground between an unlisted procedure and the detailed specifics found in most codes.

For instance, 66250 *Revision or repair of operative wound of anterior segment, any type, early or late, major or minor procedure*, covers the repair of any postoperative complication. This code is used for any complication occurring outside the global services or time frame of the original surgery. This and other nonspecific codes from the ocular section of CPT will not be listed in the body of this book, since too many variations exist to adequately describe each.

Another nonspecific code is 66940 *Removal of lens material; extracapsular (other than 66840, 66850, 66852)*. Use this if the three listed codes do not adequately describe the surgery performed. This nonspecific code will be referenced in the Comments section of similar procedures.

Two other codes deal with nonspecific methods outside of CPT descriptions. Both 67109 and 69112 report the repair of retinal detachments. If a method other than those reported in 67101–67108 and 67110 is used to repair a detached retina, report 67109. Any method of retinal repair performed as a repeat procedure is reported with 67112. Both of these codes are referenced in the Comments section of codes dealing with retinal repair.

Explanation

CPT descriptions are written for people with medical training and may not offer the details a lay person needs to choose a code based on the contents of an operative report or patient's chart. The explanations in *Coding Illustrated* are intended to describe each procedure in simple terms. Technical language that might be used by the physician is included and defined.

Because there is often more than one way to perform a procedure, *Coding Illustrated* describes the most common method, using key words commonly found in an operative report or chart. If our description varies too greatly from the operative report, another code might be more appropriate. If a satisfactory code description cannot be matched to the chart, consult the physician.

Comments

The Comments section for each code gives instruction on how the code should be applied, provides related CPT codes, and offers helpful hints concerning common billing errors associated with the code. Much of this information was drafted by consultants and other members of the technical staff at Medicode, Inc., the parent company of Med-Index Publications. Some instructions are directly from CPT.

ICD•9 Codes

ICD·9 is a systematic listing of codes that describes medical conditions. It was originally designed to track health statistics, but has become the standard mechanism for insurance payers to determine medical necessity or gauge whether a diagnosis warrants the services provided.

ICD·9 codes are published in three volumes. Volumes 1 and 2 list diagnosis codes, while Volume 3 provides inpatient procedure codes.

ICD-9 Procedural Codes

Volume 3 of ICD-9 lists procedural codes hospitals use in reporting charges to the government. In this field, we cross-referenced the CPT code to its corresponding ICD-9 Volume 3 code or codes.

ICD-9 Diagnostic Codes

Coding Illustrated teams each CPT code with the ICD·9 codes most frequently associated with that procedure in Medicode's database. These diagnosis codes are then edited by Medicode technical staff for appropriateness. Be aware that this list cannot not be inclusive of every possible diagnosis for a given procedure.

Data Table

Data appearing within the table placed in the lower left-hand portion of the two-page spread is gleaned from Medicode's database of more than 250 million medical billing entries. This data reflects what is generally considered usual and reasonable among payers, but not necessarily what is universally acceptable. Coders may want to consult individual payers for more specific information.

Follow-up Days

The global fee for most surgical procedures includes a certain number of days of postoperative follow-up care. This field lists the most commonly accepted number of follow-up days for the procedure.

When members of a code family are grouped together but information on follow-up days or anesthesia codes differs, the numerical data will be separated by a slash (/). For instance, 65270 *Repair of laceration; conjunctiva, with or without nonperforating laceration sclera, direct closure* usually has no follow-up days. This code is grouped with 65272 *...conjunctiva by mobilization and* *rearrangement, without hospitalization,* which generally requires 7 follow-up days. This difference will be shown as 0/7 in the Follow-Up Days grid.

Assist at Surgery

Some surgeries require the aid of an assistant surgeon. This field indicates whether most payers consider an assistant warranted for the procedure.

Prior Approval

Payers consider the necessity of a surgery when determining reimbursement, and in some cases must be contacted before a procedure is performed. A "Y" in the Prior Approval field identifies an invasive, elective procedure that has been frequently or is potentially overutilized and may be of questionable medical necessity. The procedure is associated with high cost and/or high volume, and generally requires prior approval by payers for reimbursement to be considered.

Anesthesia Code

The appropriate CPT anesthesia code(s) for the procedure being referenced is listed in this field. There are procedures, however, for which specific codes cannot be indicated, or anesthesia is already included in the surgery code. In these instances, abbreviated indicators appear in this field.

NA (Not Applicable): Some procedures are performed without any type of anesthesia or are performed with a local anesthetic which, by CPT definition of the global surgical package, is included with the surgery. In these cases, NA appears in this field. If circumstances require general, regional, or other supportive anesthesia services for a procedure noted with NA, report the appropriate anesthesia CPT code located by body site.

SC (Subsidiary Code): When SC appears in this field rather than an anesthesia code, the procedure is subsidiary, or secondary, to a more primary service from which the anesthesia code is determined.

SP (Surgical Procedure): SP indicates an invasive surgical procedure performed by an anesthesiologist or a certified registered nurse anesthetist, such as placing an arterial catheter. Some third-party payers calculate reimbursement for these procedures from usual, reasonable, and customary fee allowances or schedules.

BR (By Report): BR indicates a procedure with variables that make the provision of a code in this field impossible. Coding may be different for each claim and must be handled on a by-report basis. Include a special report and review of the medical documentation when filing the claim.

Should Not Be Billed

The process of coding separately the individual components of a major surgery when a single code includes those components is called "unbundling" or "fragmenting." This field lists the CPT-coded procedures that should not be broken out and reported in addition to the referenced code.

For example, 65900 reports the removal of epithelial downgrowth from the anterior chamber of the eye. Separate codes exist for direct repair of a severing adhesions in the anterior segment (65860) and for the injection of air or liquid into the anterior chamber (66020), but each service is included in 65900 and should not be reported separately.

Insurers are becoming increasingly proficient in interpreting reimbursement coding, and providers must use the most appropriate codes available.

HCPCS Level II Codes

HCPCS is an acronym (pronounced "hick-picks") for the HCFA Common Procedure Coding System. This field presents Level II (national) codes that provide a uniform method for reporting medical supplies and equipment as well as select services provided on an outpatient basis. Level II codes were developed and are maintained by the Health Care Financing Administration (HCFA) for Medicare reporting, but they are rapidly gaining recognition in the commercial payer industry. CPT codes are considered Level I codes of HCPCS.

HCFA mandates the use of HCPCS codes on Medicare claims, and many states also require them on Medicaid forms. Before applying the HCPCS Level II codes found in this book to your Medicare services, contact your carrier for a current listing of Level III (local) codes and modifiers that normally override the Level II codes.

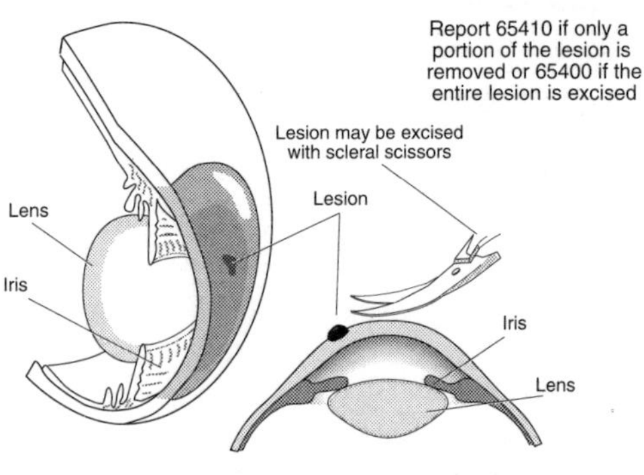

CORNEAL LESION EXCISION

The appendixes to *The Eyeball* include a listing of Level II codes possibly appropriate for those structures. In addition, several Level II modifiers are relevant to procedures involving the eyeball. Among these modifiers are:

AP Determination of refractive state was not performed in the course of diagnostic ophthalmological examination
LS FDA-monitored intraocular lens implant
LT Left side (used to indentify procedures performed on left eye)
RT Right side (used to identify procedures performed on right eye)
PL Progessive addition lenses
VP Aphakic patient

Illustrations

The illustrations that accompany the *Coding Illustrated* series provide coders a better understanding of the medical procedures referenced by the codes and data. The graphics offer coders a visual link between the technical language of the operative report and the cryptic descriptions accompanying the codes. The depictions usually include a labeled view of the affected body area, and occasionally tools and devices pertinent to the referenced procedure. Since many codes within a given set are similar in nature, graphics have been developed to highlight differences for clearer code selection.

The illustrations are almost always simplified schematic representations, oftentimes of complex and delicate medical procedures. In many instances, proper anatomical detail is given over to a clearer picture of coding the procedure. As such, only a lay knowledge of a given medical procedure can be obtained from any depiction. All graphic material was computer generated by Med-Index Publications staff. Valuable reference was drawn from a broad spectrum of surgical, clinical, and anatomic publications.

Appendixes

The goal of the *Coding Illustrated* series is to provide a single-volume, three-in-one coding reference. To keep each volume manageable, we have made them highly specific and narrowly defined. But in order to provide a complete coding guide, we have included appendixes to reference CPT codes for radiology, pathology and laboratory, and HCPCS Level II codes that may be incidental to the procedures found in the body of the volume.

Radiology Codes

In most practices, radiological services associated with the eyeball are performed at outside facilities, or the services are performed in the office but evaluated by an outside radiologist. A list of applicable CPT radiology codes and their descriptions is provided as Appendix A.

Reimbursement for radiological procedures consists of two components: the technical and the professional. The technical component is that part of the procedure specific to the equipment, including the technician. The professional component is specific to the physician's evaluation of the x-rays.

Pathology and Laboratory Codes

Most physician practices use outside laboratories to perform anything more than a rudimentary lab service. Because a number of practices do perform some of their own lab work, we have included as Appendix B a list of CPT codes for laboratory services common to the eye. Information on how the service is executed, possible drug interactions, and conditions often associated with each service is listed.

Level II HCPCS Codes

Level II HCPCS codes are used in billing Medicare and some third-party payers. The codes appearing in Appendix C are a subset of the entire list, showing only those codes most often associated with the outpatient treatment of the eye.

The first group of codes included in Appendix C is the A codes, used to report medical and surgical supplies. Next are the E codes that report durable medical equipment and the J codes assigned to drugs. V codes represent vision services.

Summary

Computer technology now allows payers to evaluate medical claims in ways that were once impossible or too time-consuming to consider. Mismatched or inappropriate codes are flagged, and the reimbursement process becomes mired in questions and correspondence that can take months to resolve. Accurate coding is more important than ever.

Coding Illustrated was developed to help providers comply with the emerging standards by which medical services are coded, reported, and paid. Remember that *Coding Illustrated* is a post-treatment medical reference, and as such it is inappropriate to use this manual to select medical treatment.

The Eyeball

CPT Description

65091 Evisceration of ocular contents; without implant

65093 with implant

Explanation

The physician removes the contents of the eyeball: the vitreous, retina, choroid, lens, iris, and ciliary muscles. Retained is the tough, white outer shell (the sclera). After an ocular speculum has been inserted, the physician dissects the conjunctiva free from the sclera. An elliptical incision is made in the sclera surrounding the cornea, and the contents of the anterior chamber of removed. The physician uses a spoon to remove the contents of the posterior chamber, and then scrapes the inside of the sclera with gauze on a curet. Only the scleral shell remains. The conjunctiva may be removed. A temporary (e.g., for 65091) or permanent (e.g., for 65093) implant is inserted into the scleral shell at this time. The sclera is attached to the implant, usually with sutures.

Comments

An implant is always placed after an evisceration to maintain the viability of the scleral shell. However, if the patient must be monitored for a period of time before an implant is permanently affixed (as in the case of infection or a malignancy), a temporary implant is used and 65091 ("without implant") is reported. Use 65093 only if the initial implant is a permanent one. See 65130 for delayed placement of the permanent artificial eye. Any rearrangement of conjunctival tissues following evisceration and the placement of a permanent artificial eye can be separately reported with 68320–68340. See 92330 and 92335 for prescription, fitting, and supply of the artificial eye.

Commonly Associated ICD•9 Procedural Codes

16.31 Removal of ocular contents with synchronous implant into scleral shell

16.39 Other evisceration of eyeball

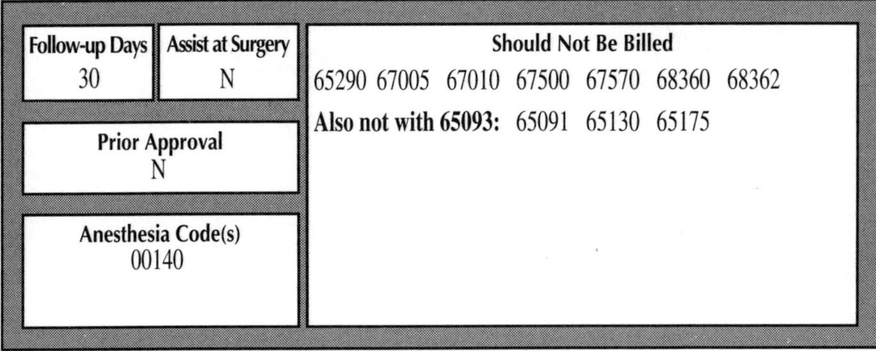

Follow-up Days	Assist at Surgery
30	N

Prior Approval
N

Anesthesia Code(s)
00140

Should Not Be Billed

65290 67005 67010 67500 67570 68360 68362

Also not with 65093: 65091 65130 65175

Commonly Associated ICD•9 Diagnostic Codes

360.41 Blind hypotensive eye
360.42 Blind hypertensive eye

Also for 65093:

V43.0 Eye globe replaced by other means
V52.2 Fitting and adjustment of artificial eye

Applicable HCPCS Level II Codes

A4305 Disposable drug delivery system, flow rate of 50 ml or greater per hour
A4306 Disposable drug delivery system, flow rate of 5 ml or less per hour
A4550 Surgical tray
V2623 Prosthetic eye, plastic, custom
V2628 Fabrication and fitting of ocular conformer
V2629 Prosthetic eye, other type

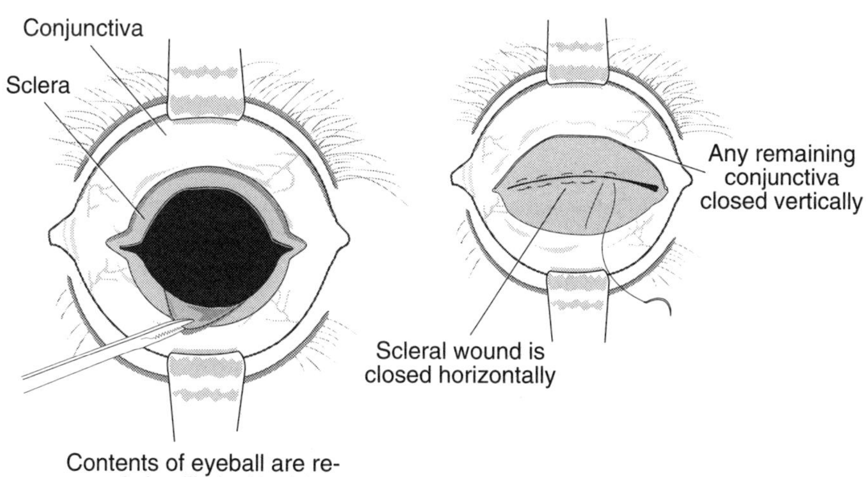

CPT Description

65101 Enucleation of eye; without implant

65103 with implant, muscles not attached to implant

65105 with implant, muscles attached to implant

Explanation

The physician severs the eyeball from the extraorbital muscles and optic nerve and removes it. After an ocular speculum has been inserted, the physician dissects the conjunctiva free at the corneal-scleral juncture (the limbus). The physician cuts each extraocular muscle at its juncture to the eyeball and severs the optic nerve. The eyeball, and sometimes the conjunctiva, is removed but the extraocular muscles remain attached at the back of the eye socket. A spherical implant is placed in the eye socket. This implant, if unattached to the extraocular muscles, may be temporary (e.g., 65101) or permanent (e.g., 65103). The extraocular muscles may be attached to the permanent implant to allow normal movement of the prosthesis (e.g., 65105).

Comments

An implant is usually placed after an enucleation. However, if the orbit must be monitored for a period of time before an implant is permanently affixed (as in the case of infection or a malignancy), a temporary implant is used and 65101 ("without implant") reported. Use 65103 or 65105 only if the initial implant is a permanent one. Any rearrangement of conjunctival tissues following enucleation and placement of an artificial eye can be separately reported with 68320–68340. Use 65135-65140 for delayed placement of a permanent artificial eyeball. See 92330 and 92335 for prescription, fitting, and supply of the artificial eye.

Commonly Associated ICD•9 Procedural Codes

16.41 Enucleation of eyeball with synchronous implant into Tenon's capsule with attachment of muscles

16.42 Enucleation of eyeball with other synchronous implant

16.49 Other enucleation of eyeball

Follow-up Days	Assist at Surgery	Should Not Be Billed
30	N	64732 64734 67500 67570 68360 68362
Prior Approval		**Also not with 65103:** 65101 65135
N		**Also not with 65105:** 65101 65103 65135 65140
Anesthesia Code(s)		
00140		

Commonly Associated ICD•9 Diagnostic Codes

190.0 Malignant neoplasm of eyeball, except conjunctiva, cornea, retina, and choroid
190.3 Malignant neoplasm of conjunctiva
190.4 Malignant neoplasm of cornea
190.5 Malignant neoplasm of retina
190.6 Malignant neoplasm of choroid
190.8 Malignant neoplasm of other specified sites of eye
360.41 Blind hypotensive eye
360.42 Blind hypertensive eye
V43.0 Eye globe replaced by other means
V52.2 Fitting and adjustment of artificial eye

Applicable HCPCS Level II Codes

A4305 Disposable drug delivery system, flow rate of 50 ml or greater per hour
A4306 Disposable drug delivery system, flow rate of 5 ml or less per hour
A4550 Surgical tray
V2623 Prosthetic eye, plastic, custom
V2628 Fabrication and fitting of ocular conformer
V2629 Prosthetic eye, other type

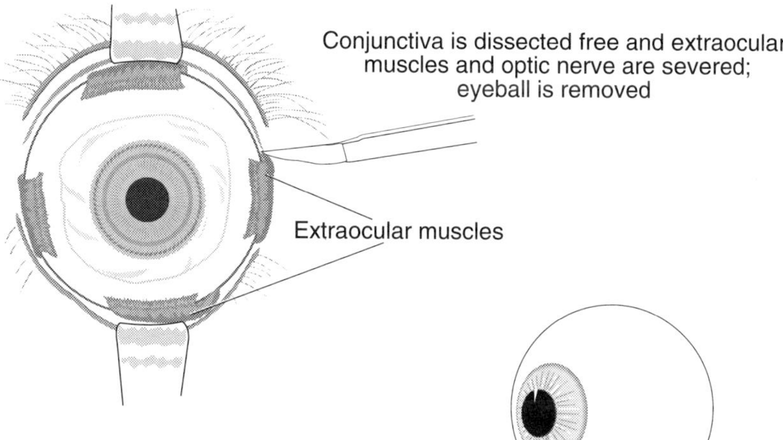

CPT Description

65110 Exenteration of orbit (does not include skin graft), removal of orbital contents; only

65112 with therapeutic removal of bone

Explanation

The physician places sutures the eyelids closed. An elliptical incision is cut through the skin, subcutaneous tissue, muscle and periosteum to the bone beginning at the upper nasal orbital rim and is carried below the brow to the lateral canthus. The incision is extended from the upper nasal quadrant along the nasal and inferior orbit rim to the lateral canthus, terminating in a wide canthotomy. The periosteum is freed around the orbital rim with a periosteum elevator, beginning in the upper temporal quadrant. The trochlea is detached with a sharp dissection. In the upper temporal quadrant, the lacrimal gland is removed. The lacrimal sac is separated from its attachments and removed. The medial and lateral canthal ligaments are cut with a blunt dissection. A blunt dissection is also used to separate the periorbita to the apex, and the firm attachment of the periosteum is cut from the bone with scissors. The orbital contents are removed. Pieces of orbital bone may be excised (e.g., for 65112). The orbit is packed with dry gauze and pressure is applied to control bleeding.

Comments

If a muscle or mycutaneous flap is created after exenteration, use 65114. For free graft to orbit (split skin) see 15120 and 15121; for free, full thickness, see 15260 and 15261. For eyelid repair involving more than skin, see 67930. For placement of a permanent orbital implant, see 67550.

Commonly Associated ICD•9 Procedural Codes

16.51 Exenteration of orbit with removal of adjacent structures

16.52 Exenteration of orbit with therapeutic removal of orbital bone

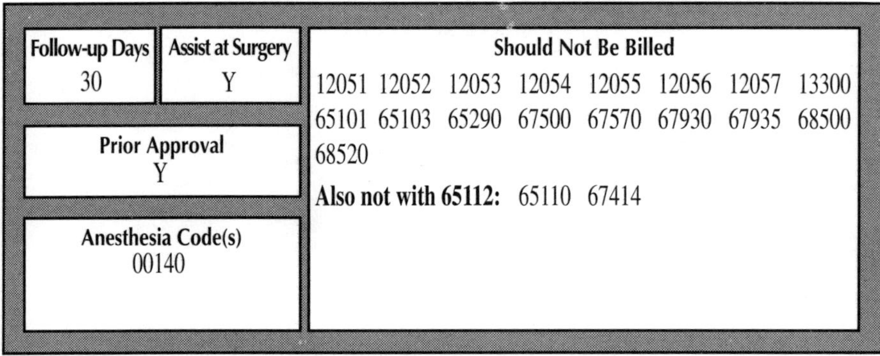

Follow-up Days	Assist at Surgery
30	Y

Prior Approval
Y

Anesthesia Code(s)
00140

Should Not Be Billed

12051 12052 12053 12054 12055 12056 12057 13300 65101 65103 65290 67500 67570 67930 67935 68500 68520

Also not with 65112: 65110 67414

Commonly Associated ICD•9 Diagnostic Codes

172.1 Malignant melanoma of skin of eyelid, including canthus
190.0 Malignant neoplasm of eyeball, except conjunctiva, cornea, retina, and choroid
190.2 Malignant neoplasm of lacrimal gland
190.3 Malignant neoplasm of conjunctiva
190.4 Malignant neoplasm of cornea
190.5 Malignant neoplasm of retina
190.6 Malignant neoplasm of choroid
190.8 Malignant neoplasm of other specified sites of eye

Applicable HCPCS Level II Codes

HCPCS Level II codes are used to report the supplies, durable medical equipment, and certain medical services provided on an outpatient basis. Because this is an inpatient procedure, no HCPCS Level II codes apply.

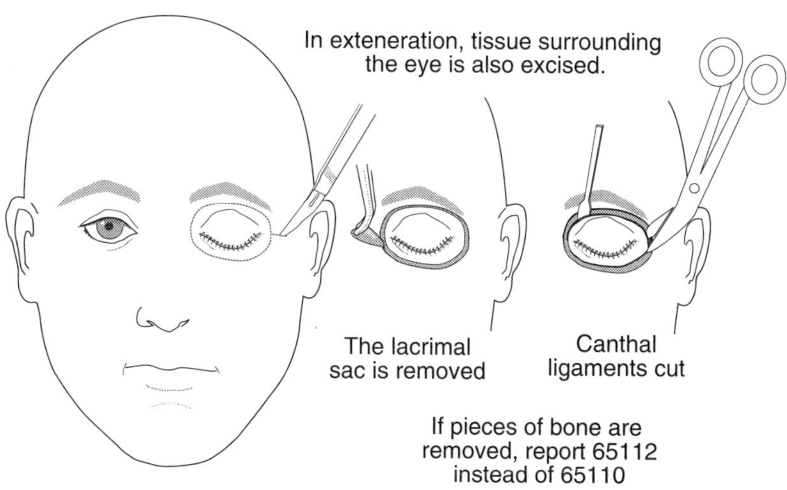

This more extensive procedure is usually reserved for malignancies

65114 CPT CODE

CPT Description

Exenteration of orbit (does not include skin graft), removal of orbital contents; with muscle or myocutaneous flap

Explanation

The physician splits the upper and lower eyelids at the gray line throughout their length, leaving the cilia and the skin anteriorly, and the tarsus, the orbicularis muscle, the conjunctiva, the palpebral muscle and the fascial planes posteriorly. The margins of the posterior halves of the lids are sutured together. The lateral bony wall and the temporal fossa are exposed by lateral canthotomy and dissection of the skin, continuous with both lids. The orbital septum is incised. The trochlea is detached with a sharp dissection. The lacrimal gland and lacrimal sac are removed. The medial and lateral canthal ligaments are cut with a blunt dissection. A blunt dissection is also used to separate the periorbita to the apex. The firm attachment of the periosteum is cut from the bone with scissors. The orbital contents are removed. An incision is made in the fascia at the origin of the temporalis muscle. Fascia and muscle are reflected from the temporal fossa. Adherent fascia is excised from the upper margin of the zygomatic process. The muscle is dissected beneath the process. The temporalis muscle and its fascia are taken through the opening into the orbit. After the muscle and the fascia are spread to fill the orbit, they are sutured to the periosteum.

Comments

If no muscle or myocutaneous flap is performed, see 65110 or 65112. The placement of a temporary orbital implant is considered incidental in this procedure.

Commonly Associated ICD•9 Procedural Codes

16.51 Exenteration of orbit with removal of adjacent structures

16.52 Exenteration of orbit with therapeutic removal of orbital bone

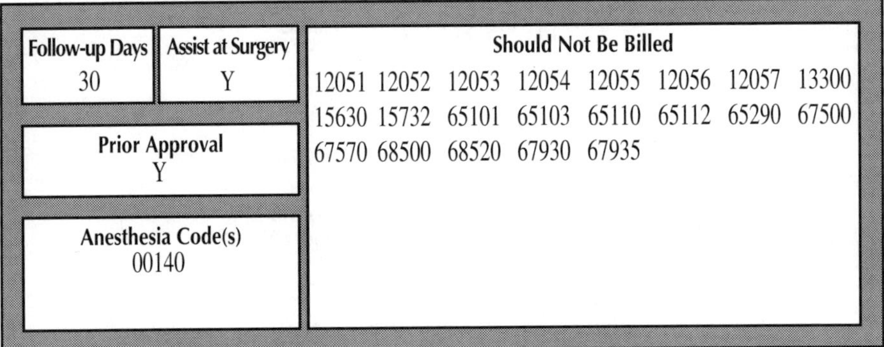

Follow-up Days	Assist at Surgery
30	Y

Prior Approval
Y

Anesthesia Code(s)
00140

Should Not Be Billed

12051	12052	12053	12054	12055	12056	12057	13300
15630	15732	65101	65103	65110	65112	65290	67500
67570	68500	68520	67930	67935			

Commonly Associated ICD•9 Diagnostic Codes

172.1 Malignant melanoma of skin of eyelid, including canthus
190.0 Malignant neoplasm of eyeball, except conjunctiva, cornea, retina, and choroid
190.2 Malignant neoplasm of lacrimal gland
190.3 Malignant neoplasm of conjunctiva
190.4 Malignant neoplasm of cornea
190.5 Malignant neoplasm of retina
190.6 Malignant neoplasm of choroid
190.8 Malignant neoplasm of other specified sites of eye

Applicable HCPCS Level II Codes

HCPCS Level II codes are used to report the supplies, durable medical equipment, and certain medical services provided on an outpatient basis. Because this is an inpatient procedure, no HCPCS Level II codes apply.

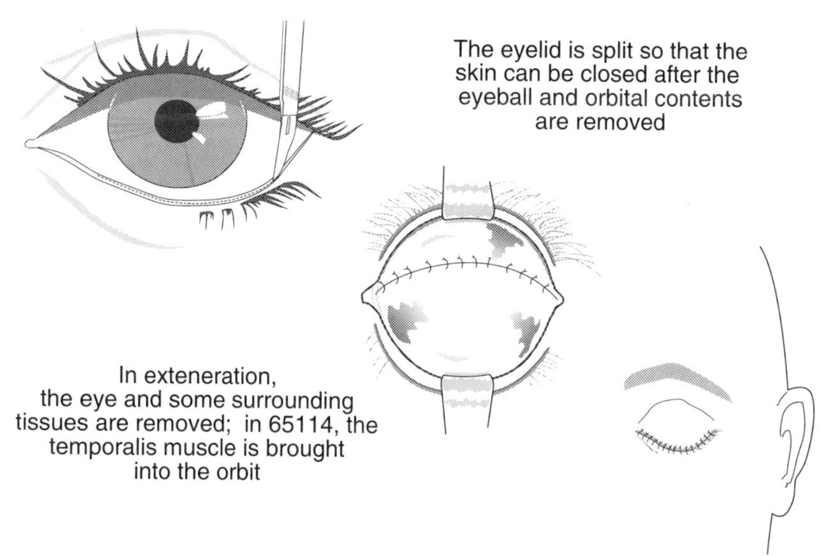

65125 CPT CODE

CPT Description

Modification of ocular implant (eg, drilling receptacle for prosthesis appendage) (separate procedure)

Explanation

The physician modifies an ocular implant that has been created elsewhere. The modifications may include the addition of screws or other prosthetic appendages to alter the shape of the prosthesis so that it better fits the patient's eye. The physician may drill holes to accommodate the screws.

Comments

Note that 65125 is a separate procedure, and as such, is usually a component of the insertion or the reinsertion of an ocular implant and is usually not reported separately. However, if modification of the ocular implant alone is performed, use 65125. See 92330 and 92335 for prescription, fitting, and supply of an artificial eye.

Commonly Associated ICD•9 Procedural Codes

95.34 Ocular prosthetics

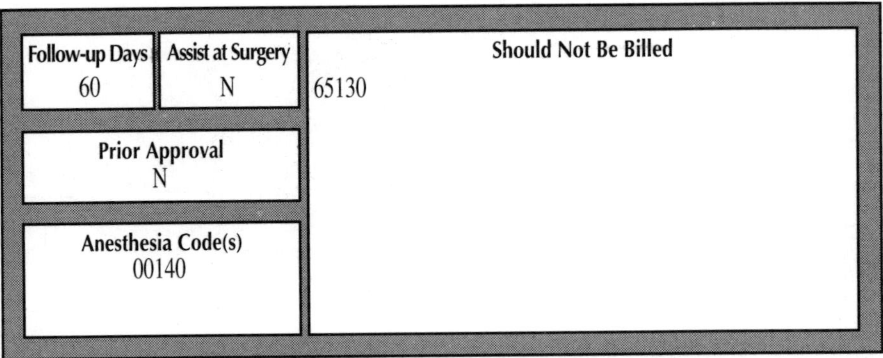

Follow-up Days	Assist at Surgery	Should Not Be Billed
60	N	65130

Prior Approval
N

Anesthesia Code(s)
00140

Commonly Associated ICD•9 Diagnostic Codes

996.59 Mechanical complication of other implant and internal device, not elsewhere classified

V10.84 Personal history of malignant neoplasm of eye

V52.2 Fitting and adjustment of artificial eye

Applicable HCPCS Level II Codes

L8610 Ocular prosthesis

V2625 Enlargement of ocular prosthesis

V2626 Reduction of ocular prosthesis

V2628 Fabrication and fitting of ocular conformer

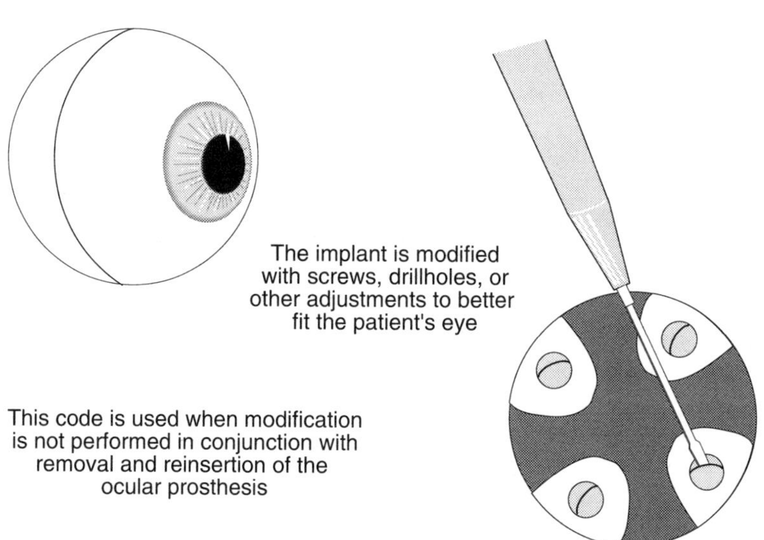

CPT Description

65130 Insertion of ocular implant secondary; after evisceration, in scleral shell

65135 after enucleation, muscles not attached to implant

65140 after enucleation, muscles attached to implant

Explanation

The physician inserts a permanent ocular prosthesis into a patient's orbit. In each case, an ocular speculum is placed in the eye, any conjunctiva is retracted, and any temporary prosthesis is removed. In a patient whose eye has been eviscerated, the implant is attached to the remaining sclera (e.g., 65130). In a patient following enucleation, the implant is otherwise secured (e.g., 65135). In some cases, eye muscles are attached to corresponding niches in the prosthesis to provide for more natural movement of the artificial eye following enucleation (e.g., 65140).

Comments

See 92330 or 92335 for prescription, fitting, and supply of an artificial eye. If the implant is placed secondary to enucleation, report 65103 or 65105 instead. Any rearrangement of conjunctival tissues and placement of an artificial eye can be separately reported with 68320–68340. For orbital implant insertion, see 67550.

Commonly Associated ICD•9 Procedural Codes

16.61 Secondary insertion of ocular implant

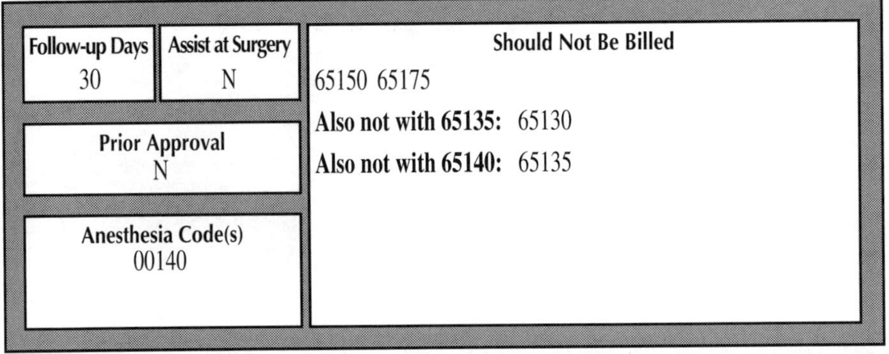

Follow-up Days	Assist at Surgery
30	N

Prior Approval
N

Anesthesia Code(s)
00140

Should Not Be Billed

65150 65175

Also not with 65135: 65130

Also not with 65140: 65135

Commonly Associated ICD•9 Diagnostic Codes

V10.84 Personal history of malignant neoplasm of eye
V43.0 Eye globe replaced by other means
V52.2 Fitting and adjustment of artificial eye

Applicable HCPCS Level II Codes

A4305 Disposable drug delivery system, flow rate of 50 ml or greater per hour
A4306 Disposable drug delivery system, flow rate of 5 ml or less per hour
A4550 Surgical tray
L8610 Ocular prosthesis
V2623 Prosthetic eye, plastic, custom
V2628 Fabrication and fitting of ocular conformer
V2629 Prosthetic eye, other type

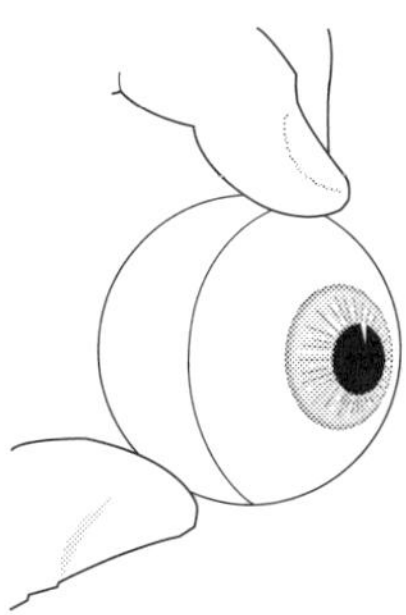

The implant is attached to the sclera of an eviscerated eye in 65130

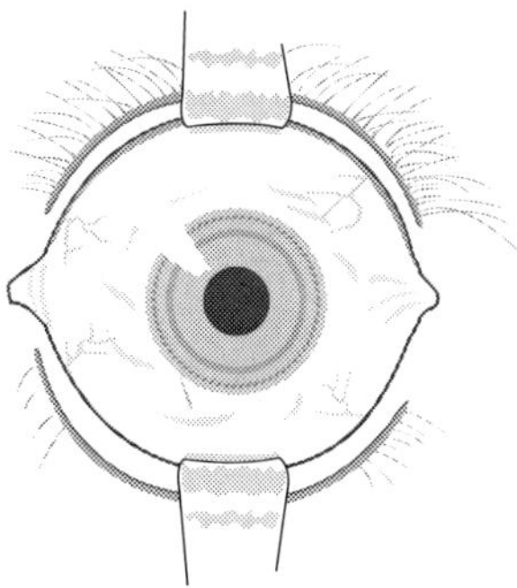

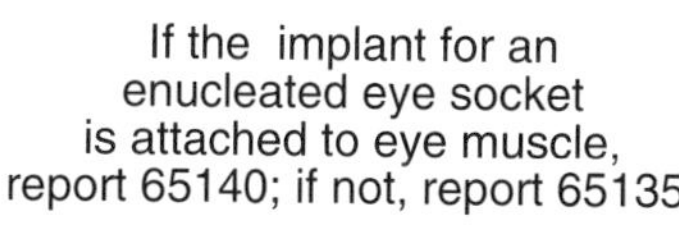

If the implant for an enucleated eye socket is attached to eye muscle, report 65140; if not, report 65135

CPT Description

65150 Reinsertion of ocular implant; with or without conjunctival graft

65155 with use of foreign material for reinforcement and/or attachment of muscles to implant

Explanation

The physician returns an ocular prosthesis to the patient's eye socket. After an ocular speculum is inserted, the physician places the ocular prosthesis back into an eye from which it had been previously removed. The prosthesis is attached to the sclera in an eviscerated eye, or otherwise secured in an enucleated eye (e.g., 65150). In 65155, foreign material may be required to better secure the prosthesis and/or the prosthesis may be reattached to extraocular muscles. In either procedure, conjunctival tissue may be grafted over the prosthesis once it is secured.

Comments

For orbital implant insertion, see 67550.

Commonly Associated ICD•9 Procedural Codes

10.42 Reconstruction of conjunctival cul-de-sac with free graft

10.43 Other reconstruction of conjunctival cul-de-sac

16.61 Secondary insertion of ocular implant

16.62 Revision and reinsertion of ocular implant

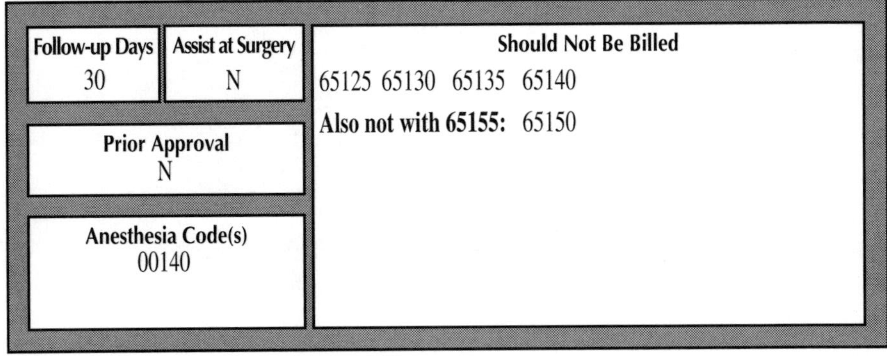

Follow-up Days	Assist at Surgery	Should Not Be Billed
30	N	65125 65130 65135 65140
Prior Approval		**Also not with 65155:** 65150
N		
Anesthesia Code(s)		
00140		

Commonly Associated ICD•9 Diagnostic Codes

V10.84 Personal history of malignant neoplasm of eye
V52.2 Fitting and adjustment of artificial eye

Applicable HCPCS Level II Codes

A4305 Disposable drug delivery system, flow rate of 50 ml or greater per hour
A4306 Disposable drug delivery system, flow rate of 5 ml or less per hour
A4550 Surgical tray
L8610 Ocular prosthesis
V2623 Prosthetic eye, plastic, custom
V2628 Fabrication and fitting of ocular conformer
V2629 Prosthetic eye, other type

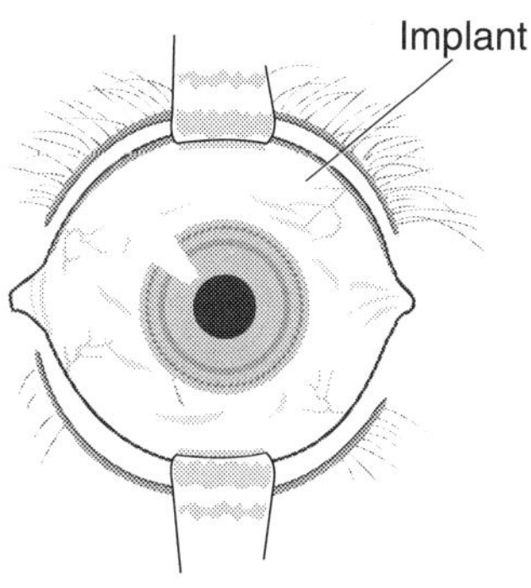

In an eviscerated eye, the implant is attached to the sclera and in the enucleated eye it is attached to the extraocular eye muscles; in either case, 65150 is reported

Report 65150 for reinsertion of an implant in an enucleated eye; if foreign material is used to secure the prosthesis, use 65155

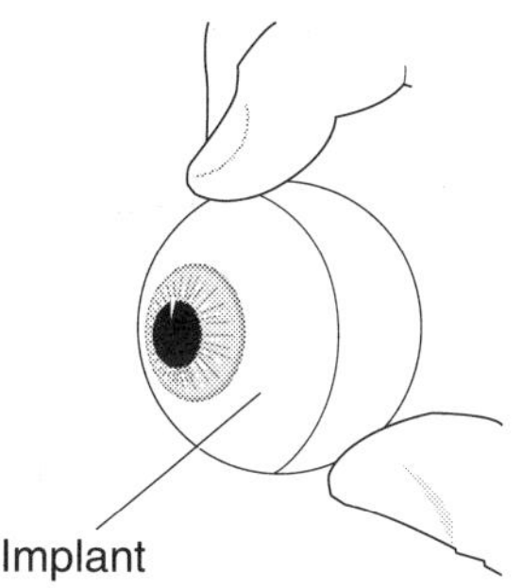

65175 CPT CODE

CPT Description

Removal of ocular implant

Explanation

The physician removes the ocular implant from the eye socket. After placing an ocular speculum, the physician cuts and retracts any conjunctival tissue or Tenon's capsule overlying the prosthesis. Any connection between the implant and extraocular muscle or sclera is severed and the ocular implant is removed.

Comments

An ocular implant is inside, and an orbital implant is outside, the muscular cone. For removal of orbital implant, use 67560.

Commonly Associated ICD•9 Procedural Codes

16.71 Removal of ocular implant

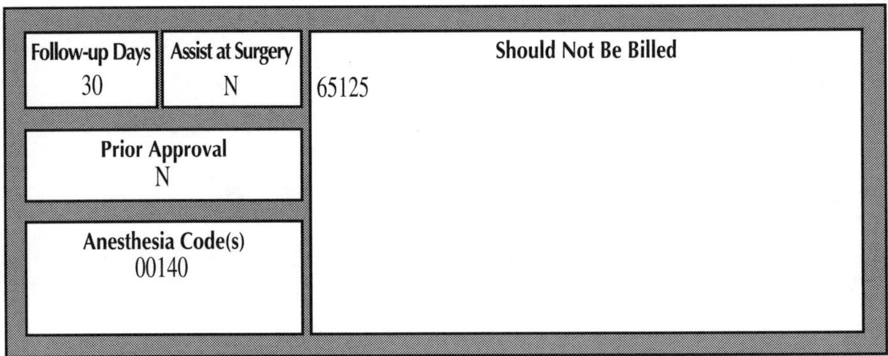

Follow-up Days	Assist at Surgery	Should Not Be Billed
30	N	65125
Prior Approval		
N		
Anesthesia Code(s)		
00140		

Commonly Associated ICD•9 Diagnostic Codes

376.00 Acute inflammation of orbit, unspecified
376.10 Chronic inflammation of orbit, unspecified
379.91 Pain in or around eye
996.59 Mechanical complication of other implant and internal device, not elsewhere classified
996.69 Infection and inflammatory reaction due to other internal prosthetic device, implant, and graft

Applicable HCPCS Level II Codes

A4305 Disposable drug delivery system, flow rate of 50 ml or greater per hour
A4306 Disposable drug delivery system, flow rate of 5 ml or less per hour
A4550 Surgical tray
V2623 Prosthetic eye, plastic, custom
V2628 Fabrication and fitting of ocular conformer
V2629 Prosthetic eye, other type

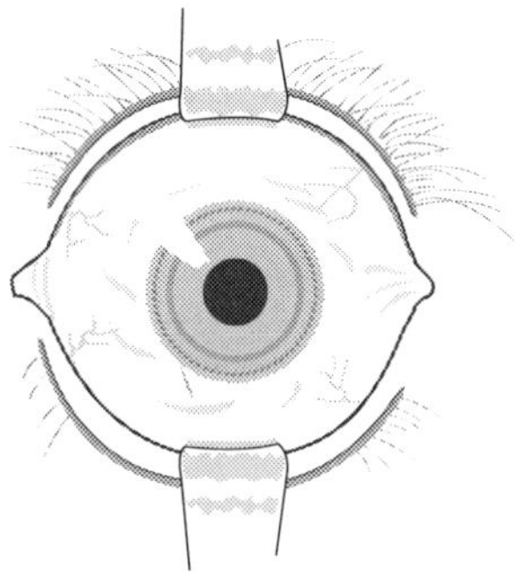

An ocular speculum helps the physician access the prothesis. Any attachments are severed

The implant may be removed from an eviscerated or enucleated eye

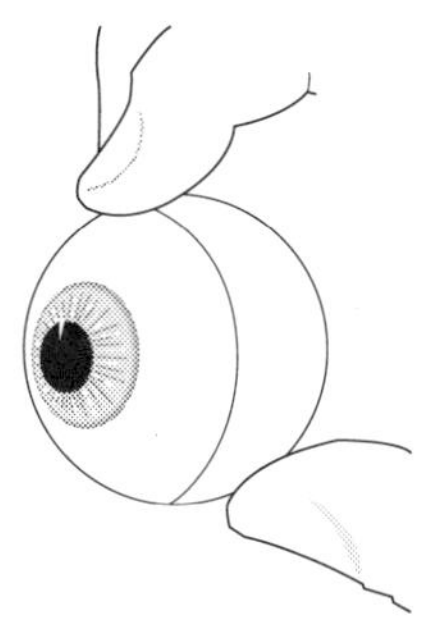

65205*–65210* CPT CODES

CPT Description

65205 Removal of foreign body, external eye; conjunctival superficial

65210 conjunctival embedded (includes concretions), subconjunctival, or scleral nonperforating

Explanation

The physician picks the foreign body or mineral deposit from the conjunctiva with the side of the beveled edge of a needle (e.g., 65205). A small incision may be required to remove an embedded foreign body (e.g., 65210). In this case, the physician may cut a V-shaped incision to access the defect through a flap, or a straight incision may be made. The incision may penetrate the conjunctiva, but it does not penetrate the sclera. Generally, a slit lamp is used when removing any embedded foreign body. After the removal, the physician may apply a broad spectrum antibiotic and a moderate pressure patch over the closed lid for 24-48 hours.

Comments

Note that no repair takes place here. If a repair is made to the conjunctiva, see 65270. These procedures are usually performed without anesthesia, but topical anesthetic may be used. For removal of foreign body embedded in eyelid, see 67938. Also, these codes are accompanied by stars, and therefore describe the surgical procedure only. If other services are provided at the same time, code them separately.

Commonly Associated ICD•9 Procedural Codes

10.0 Removal of embedded foreign body from conjunctiva by incision

98.21 Removal of superficial foreign body from eye without incision

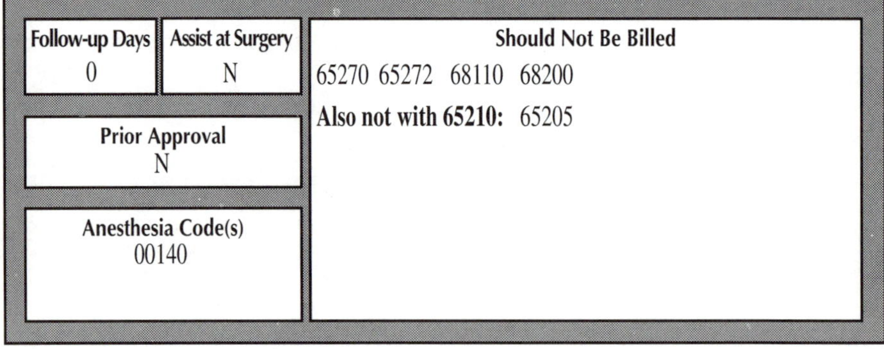

Follow-up Days	Assist at Surgery
0	N

Prior Approval
N

Anesthesia Code(s)
00140

Should Not Be Billed

65270 65272 68110 68200

Also not with 65210: 65205

Commonly Associated ICD•9 Diagnostic Codes

918.2 Superficial injury of conjunctiva
918.9 Other and unspecified superficial injuries of eye
930.1 Foreign body in conjunctival sac
930.8 Foreign body in other and combined sites on external eye

Applicable HCPCS Level II Codes

A4550 Surgical tray

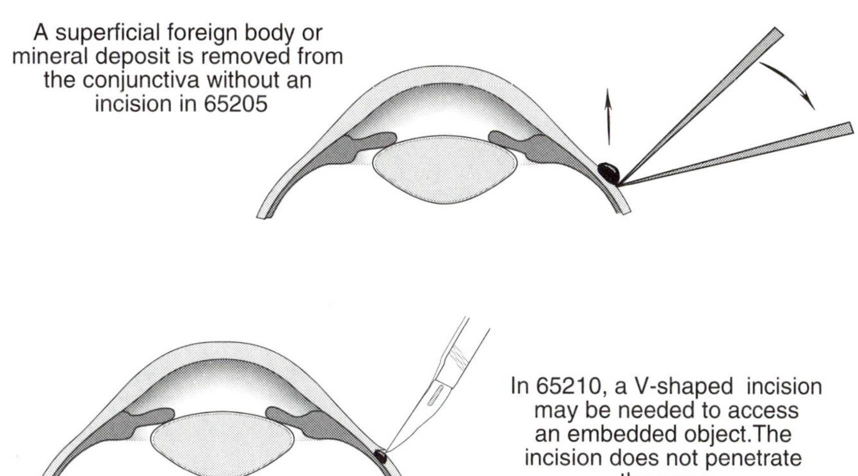

CPT Description

65220 Removal of foreign body, external eye; corneal, without slit lamp

65222 corneal, with slit lamp

Explanation

The physician may remove a superficial foreign body or mineral deposit from the cornea with the side of the beveled edge of a needle (e.g., 65220). An incision may be required to remove an embedded foreign body (e.g., 65222). If so, the physician may cut a V-shaped incision to access the defect through a flap, or a straight incision may be made. The incision does not penetrate the cornea. Generally, a slit lamp is used with any embedded foreign body. After the removal, the physician may apply a broad spectrum antibiotic and a moderate pressure patch over the closed lid for 24-48 hours.

Comments

Note that no repair takes place here. If a repair is made to the cornea, see 65275. This procedure is usually performed without anesthesia, but topical anesthetic may be used. Also, this code is accompanied by a star, and therefore describes the surgical procedure only. If other services are provided during the same medical encounter, code them separately.

Commonly Associated ICD•9 Procedural Codes

11.1 Incision of cornea

98.21 Removal of superficial foreign body from eye without incision

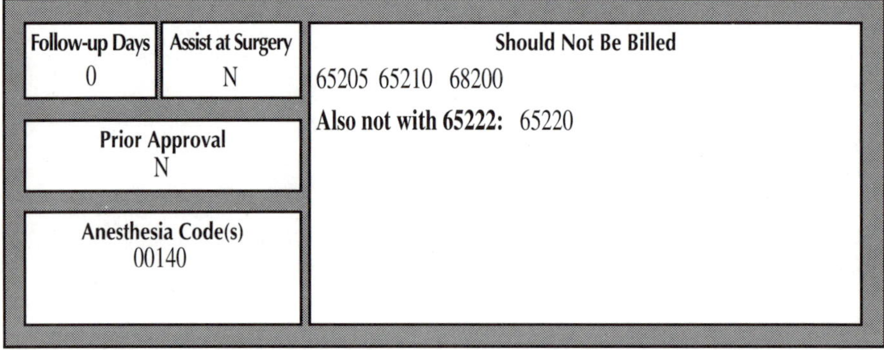

Follow-up Days	Assist at Surgery	Should Not Be Billed
0	N	65205 65210 68200
Prior Approval		**Also not with 65222:** 65220
N		
Anesthesia Code(s)		
00140		

Commonly Associated ICD•9 Diagnostic Codes

918.1 Superficial injury of cornea
918.9 Other and unspecified superficial injuries of eye
930.8 Foreign body in other and combined sites on external eye

Applicable HCPCS Level II Codes

A4550 Surgical tray

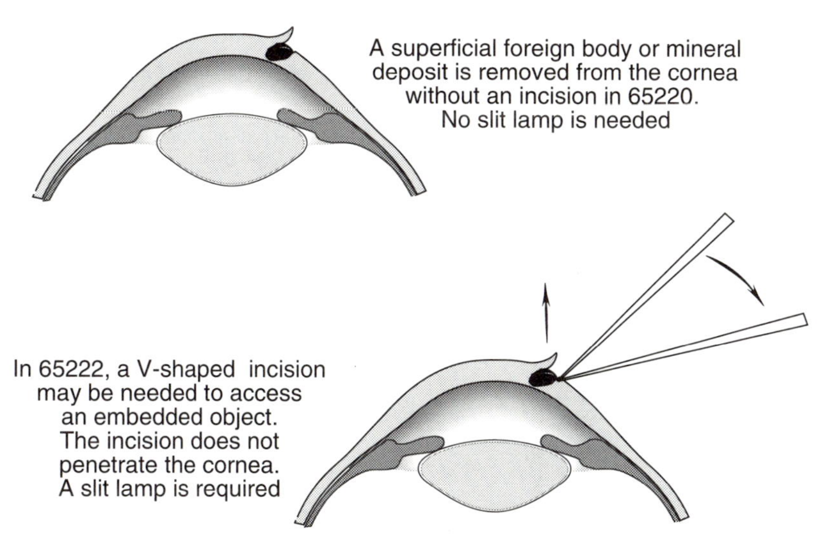

65235 CPT CODE

CPT Description

Removal of foreign body, intraocular; from anterior chamber or lens

Explanation

The anterior chamber is the area behind the cornea and in front of the iris. The physician makes a small incision in the connective tissue between the cornea and the sclera (the limbus) and retrieves the foreign body through that opening with intraocular forceps or another small instrument. Generally, foreign bodies that pierce the lens are self-sealing and removal is not attempted. The incision is sutured. The physician applies an antibiotic ointment. Sometimes a pressure patch is placed on the eye for 24-48 hours.

Comments

For diagnostic x-ray of foreign body, use 70030; for diagnostic echography, 76529; for diagnostic CT, use 70480. This procedure is generally performed with a subconjunctival or retrobulbar injection rather than general anesthesia. If the foreign body penetrates the lens and the lens itself is removed, report the lensectomy with 66840–66984. For removal of implanted material from anterior segment, see 65920. For revision or repair of operative wound of anterior segment, any type, early or late, major or minor procedure, see 66250.

Commonly Associated ICD•9 Procedural Codes

12.00 Removal of intraocular foreign body from anterior segment of eye, not otherwise specified

12.02 Removal of intraocular foreign body from anterior segment of eye without use of magnet

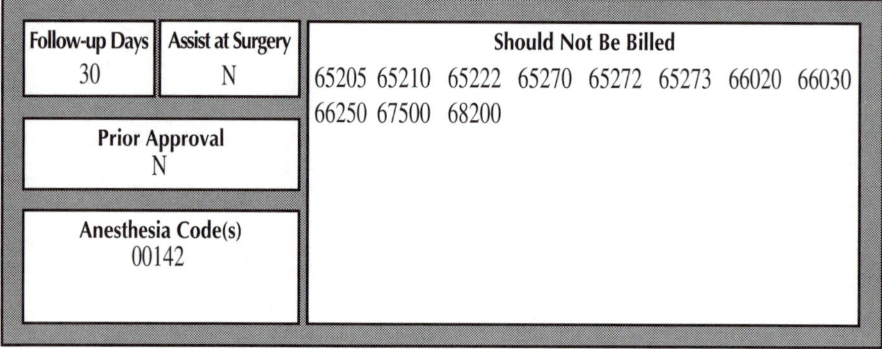

Follow-up Days	Assist at Surgery
30	N

Prior Approval
N

Anesthesia Code(s)
00142

Should Not Be Billed
65205 65210 65222 65270 65272 65273 66020 66030 66250 67500 68200

Commonly Associated ICD•9 Diagnostic Codes

360.60 Foreign body, intraocular, unspecified
360.61 Foreign body in anterior chamber
360.62 Foreign body in iris or ciliary body
364.00 Acute and subacute iridocyclitis, unspecified
364.53 Pigmentary iris degeneration
871.6 Penetration of eyeball with (nonmagnetic) foreign body

Applicable HCPCS Level II Codes

A4550 Surgical tray

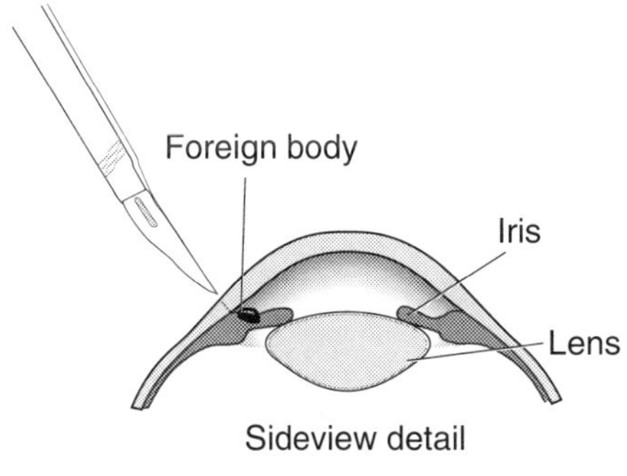

The physician removes a nonmetallic foreign body from the anterior chamber

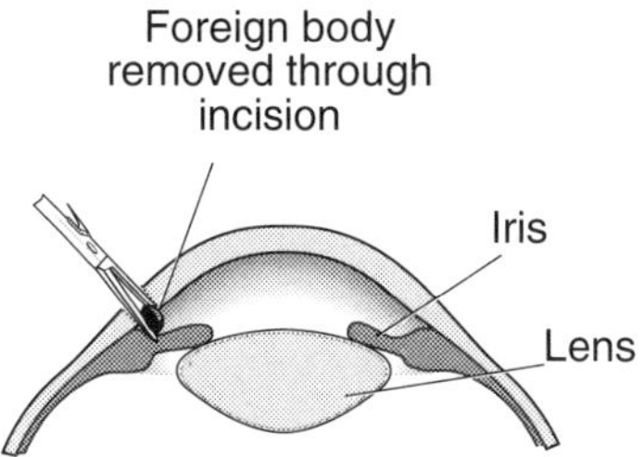

The incision is closed with sutures

65260 CPT CODE

CPT Description

Removal of foreign body, intraocular; from posterior segment, magnetic extraction, anterior or posterior route

Explanation

Diagnostic tests locate the foreign body before surgery is attempted. The physician will use an electromagnetic or magnetic probe to retrieve a metallic foreign body from the area behind the lens (the posterior segment). In the anterior route, the physician first dilates the patient's pupil. In a series of moves aligning the magnet to the metallic foreign body, the physician draws the foreign body to the front of the eye and around the lens into the anterior chamber. The physician then makes an incision in the connective tissue between the cornea and the sclera (the limbus) and retrieves the foreign body. In the posterior route, the physician makes a small incision in the conjunctiva over the site of the foreign body. A magnet is applied and the foreign body removed. The incision from either is repaired, and an injection may be required to reestablish proper fluid levels in the anterior and/or posterior chamber of the eye. A broad spectrum antibiotic or a pressure patch may be applied. Among the tools common to this procedure are Gruning's, Haab's, or Hirschberg's magnets.

Comments

For diagnostic x-ray of foreign body, use 70030; for diagnostic echography, 76529; for diagnostic CT, use 70480. Patient may be followed with serial electroretinography (92275) to ascertain function of retina prior to removal of foreign body. This procedure may be performed with a subconjunctival or retrobulbar injection rather than general anesthesia. For removal of implanted material from the posterior segment, see 67120–67121.

Commonly Associated ICD•9 Procedural Codes

14.01 Removal of foreign body from posterior segment of eye with use of magnet

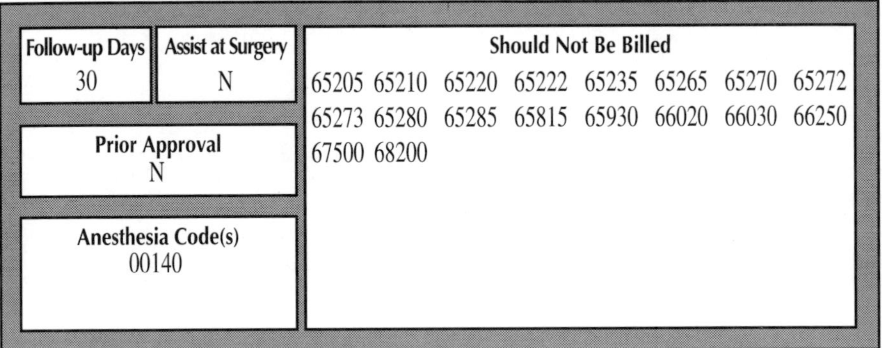

Follow-up Days	Assist at Surgery
30	N

Prior Approval
N

Anesthesia Code(s)
00140

Should Not Be Billed

65205 65210 65220 65222 65235 65265 65270 65272
65273 65280 65285 65815 65930 66020 66030 66250
67500 68200

Commonly Associated ICD•9 Diagnostic Codes

360.50 Foreign body, magnetic, intraocular, unspecified
360.53 Foreign body, magnetic, in lens
360.54 Foreign body, magnetic, in vitreous
360.55 Foreign body, magnetic, in posterior wall
360.59 Intraocular foreign body, magnetic, in other or multiple sites
364.00 Acute and subacute iridocyclitis, unspecified
364.53 Pigmentary iris degeneration
871.5 Penetration of eyeball with magnetic foreign body

Applicable HCPCS Level II Codes

HCPCS Level II codes are used to report the supplies, durable medical equipment, and certain medical services provided on an outpatient basis. This procedure can be done inpatient or in an outpatient facility; therefore, no HCPCS Level II codes apply.

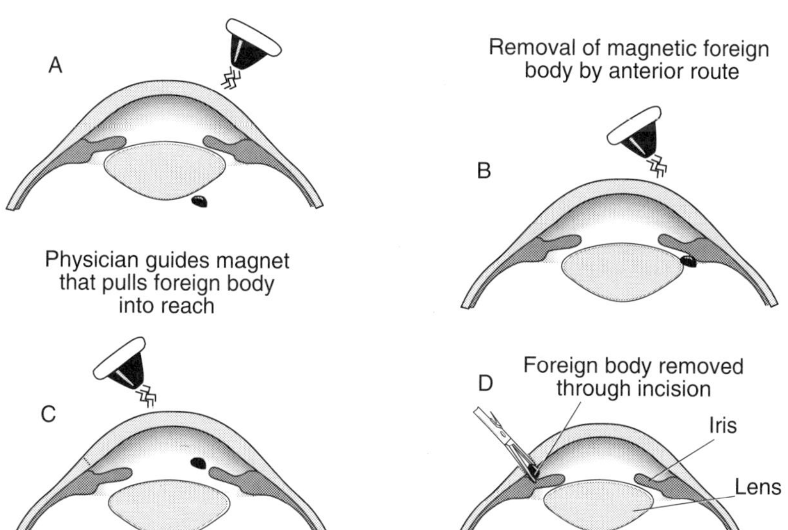

FOREIGN BODY EXTRACTION

65265 CPT CODE

CPT Description

Removal of foreign body, intraocular; from posterior segment, nonmagnetic extraction

Explanation

Diagnostic tests locate the foreign body before surgery is attempted. The physician will use intraocular forceps to retrieve the nonmetallic foreign body from the area behind the lens (the posterior segment). The physician makes an incision through the conjunctiva overlying the site of the foreign body. The foreign body is retrieved with intraocular forceps. Nonmetallic foreign bodies in the vitreous or retina may be removed through a pars plana approach. Either incision is repaired with a layered closure, and an injection may be required to reestablish proper fluid levels in the anterior or posterior chambers of eye. A broad spectrum antibiotic or a pressure patch may be applied.

Comments

For diagnostic x-ray of foreign body, use 70030; for diagnostic echography, 76529; for diagnostic CT, use 70480. This procedure is generally performed with a subconjunctival or retrobulbar injection rather than general anesthesia. For removal of an implanted lens from the posterior segment, see 67120.

Commonly Associated ICD•9 Procedural Codes

14.00 Removal of foreign body from posterior segment of eye, not otherwise specified

14.02 Removal of foreign body from posterior segment of eye without use of magnet

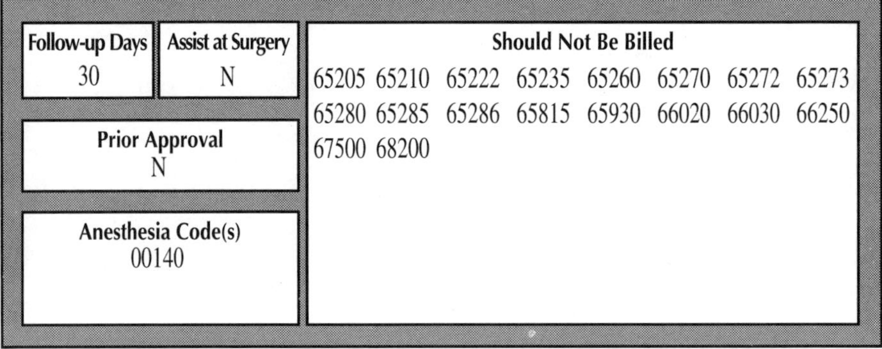

Follow-up Days	Assist at Surgery
30	N

Prior Approval
N

Anesthesia Code(s)
00140

Should Not Be Billed

65205 65210 65222 65235 65260 65270 65272 65273
65280 65285 65286 65815 65930 66020 66030 66250
67500 68200

Commonly Associated ICD•9 Diagnostic Codes

360.63 Foreign body in lens
360.64 Foreign body in vitreous
360.65 Foreign body in posterior wall of eye
360.69 Intraocular foreign body in other or multiple sites
870.4 Penetrating wound of orbit with foreign body
871.6 Penetration of eyeball with (nonmagnetic) foreign body

Applicable HCPCS Level II Codes

A4305 Disposable drug delivery system, flow rate of 50 ml or greater per hour
A4306 Disposable drug delivery system, flow rate of 5 ml or less per hour
A4550 Surgical tray

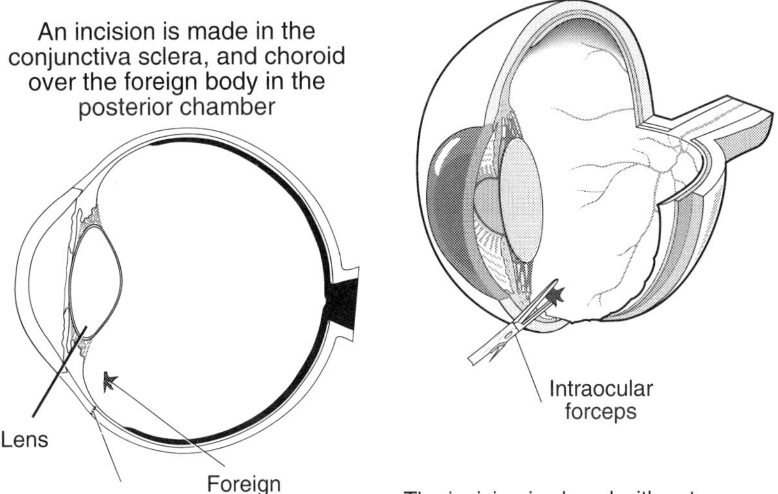

65270*–65273 CPT CODES

CPT Description

65270 Repair of laceration; conjunctiva, with or without nonperforating laceration sclera, direct closure

65272 conjunctiva, by mobilization and rearrangement, without hospitalization

65273 conjunctiva, by mobilization and rearrangement, with hospitalization

Explanation

An ocular speculum may be placed in the patient's eye. The physician irrigates the laceration and sutures the conjunctival wound (e.g., 65270). In mobilization and rearrangement (e.g., 65272), an extensive conjunctival laceration requires the creation of a flap or graft sutured over the wound, and the eyes are patched to limit their movement while the injury heals. A graft may be obtained from conjunctival tissue of the upper eyelid or from a sliding flap formed following a circumcorneal incision. Extensive repair or repair of the eye of a child may require hospitalization to further limit eye movement (e.g., 65273).

Comments

An ophthalmic exam to rule out retinal problems is usually performed in conjunction with this procedure, and is separately reported. For repair of a wound of eyelid that doesn't involve reconstructive surgery and is limited to the skin, see 12011-12018; 12051-12057; or 13150–13300. This procedure is generally performed with a subconjunctival injection or local anesthesic rather than general anesthesia.

Commonly Associated ICD•9 Procedural Codes

10.6 Repair of laceration of conjunctiva

12.81 Suture of laceration of sclera

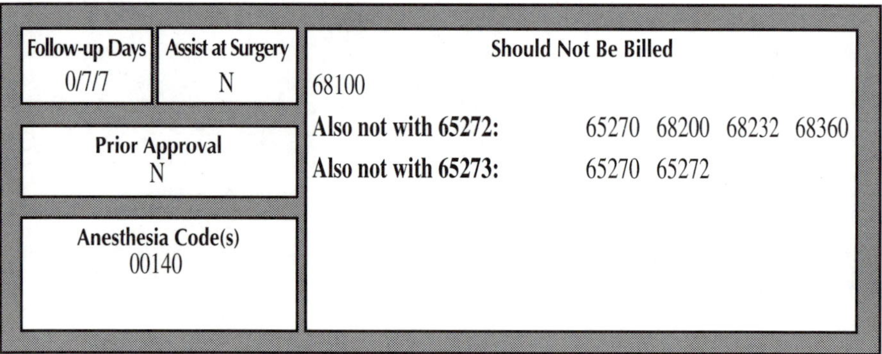

Follow-up Days	Assist at Surgery
0/7/7	N

Prior Approval
N

Anesthesia Code(s)
00140

Should Not Be Billed

68100

Also not with 65272: 65270 68200 68232 68360

Also not with 65273: 65270 65272

Commonly Associated ICD•9 Diagnostic Codes

871.0 Ocular laceration without prolapse of intraocular tissue
871.9 Unspecified open wound of eyeball
918.2 Superficial injury of conjunctiva

Also for 65272
871.4 Unspecified laceration of eye

Applicable HCPCS Level II Codes

A4550 Surgical tray

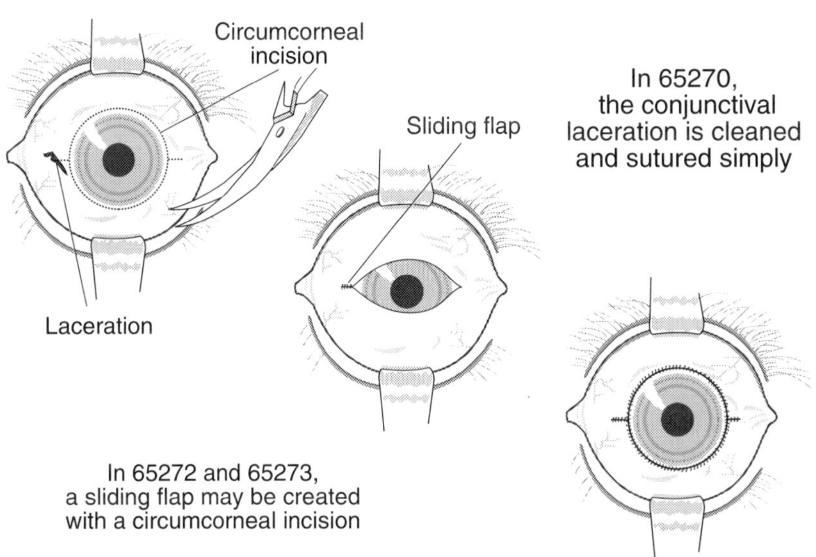

CPT Description

65275 Repair of laceration; cornea, nonperforating, with or without removal foreign body

65280 cornea and/or sclera, perforating, not involving uveal tissue

65285 cornea and/or sclera, perforating, with reposition or resection of uveal tissue

Explanation

The physician removes any foreign body from the cornea with a hollow needle or forceps and the wound is irrigated. The nonperforating tear in the cornea (e.g., 65275) is repaired with sutures. In 65280 and 65285, the perforating tear in the cornea and any tear in the sclera may be sutured. The cornea may be splinted using a soft contact lens bandage. An air or saline injection may be required to reestablish proper ocular pressure in the anterior chamber. If the laceration involves the uveal tissue (the vascular layer beneath the sclera), injured tissue may be cut out or repositioned before the uvea is sutured (e.g., 65285), and the sclera and conjunctiva may each require separate closure. In any of the three procedures, topical antibiotic or a pressure patch may be applied.

Comments

If a therapeutic contact lens is applied, it can be reported separately with 92070. This procedure is generally performed with topical anesthetic, a subconjunctival injection, or retrobulbar injection rather than general anesthesia. Repair of the laceration includes any use of a conjunctival flap or restoration of the anterior chamber by air or saline injection. For repair of iris or ciliary body, see 66680.

Commonly Associated ICD•9 Procedural Codes

11.51 Suture of corneal laceration

11.53 Repair of corneal laceration or wound with conjunctival flap

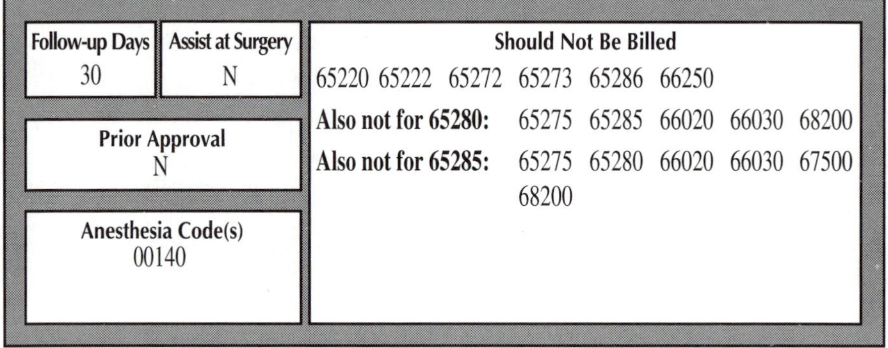

Follow-up Days	Assist at Surgery
30	N

Prior Approval
N

Anesthesia Code(s)
00140

Should Not Be Billed

65220 65222 65272 65273 65286 66250

Also not for 65280: 65275 65285 66020 66030 68200

Also not for 65285: 65275 65280 66020 66030 67500 68200

Commonly Associated ICD•9 Diagnostic Codes

871.0 Ocular laceration without prolapse of intraocular tissue
871.4 Unspecified laceration of eye
918.1 Superficial injury of cornea
930.0 Corneal foreign body
930.1 Foreign body in conjunctival sac
930.8 Foreign body in other and combined sites on external eye

Also with 65280:
871.7 Unspecified ocular penetration
871.9 Unspecified open wound of eyeball

Applicable HCPCS Level II Codes

A4305 Disposable drug delivery system, flow rate of 50 ml or greater per hour
A4306 Disposable drug delivery system, flow rate of 5 ml or less per hour
A4550 Surgical tray

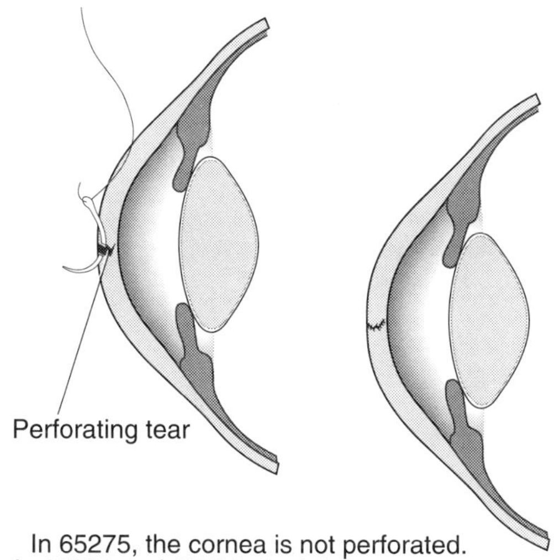

In 65275, the cornea is not perforated.
In 65280 and 65285, the injury penetrates the full corneal thickness

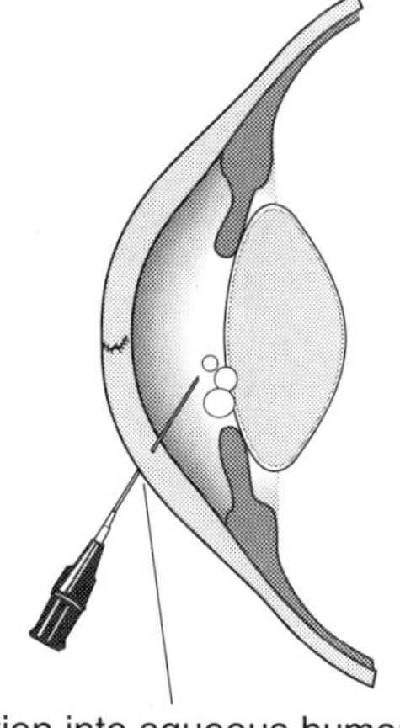

65286 CPT CODE

CPT Description

Repair of laceration; application of tissue glue, wounds of cornea and/or sclera

Explanation

Tissue glue, also called medical adhesive or Cyanoacrylate tissue adhesive, acts as a suture in laceration repairs of the cornea and/or sclera. If the cornea is perforated, the physician may seal the perforation with tissue adhesive after debriding the outermost layer of cornea (the epithelium) to enhance adhesion. The patient may be fitted with a soft contact lens to be worn during the healing process. Antibiotic ointment is applied. A pressure patch may be used.

Comments

If a therapeutic contact lens is applied, it can be reported separately using 92070. For repair of a perforating injury to the cornea without application of tissue glue, see 65280 and 65285. Repair of the laceration includes use of a conjunctival flap and any air or saline injection for restoration of fluid pressure in the anterior chamber.

Commonly Associated ICD•9 Procedural Codes

11.59 Other repair of cornea
12.89 Other operations on sclera

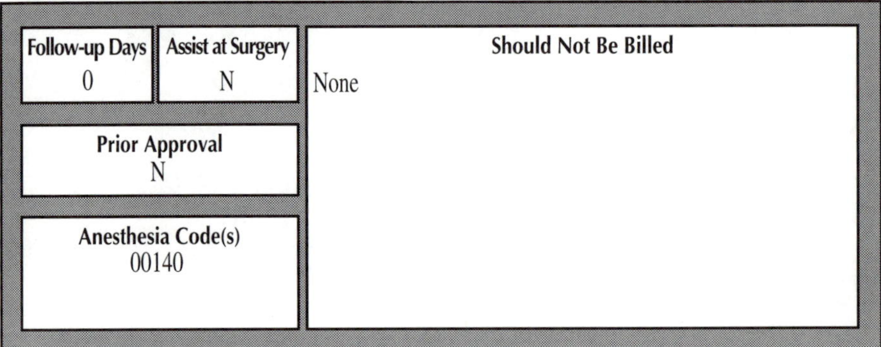

Follow-up Days	Assist at Surgery	Should Not Be Billed
0	N	None
Prior Approval N		
Anesthesia Code(s) 00140		

Commonly Associated ICD•9 Diagnostic Codes

871.0 Ocular laceration without prolapse of intraocular tissue
871.1 Ocular laceration with prolapse or exposure of intraocular tissue
871.4 Unspecified laceration of eye
918.1 Superficial injury of cornea

Applicable HCPCS Level II Codes

A4305 Disposable drug delivery system, flow rate of 50 ml or greater per hour
A4306 Disposable drug delivery system, flow rate of 5 ml or less per hour
A4550 Surgical tray

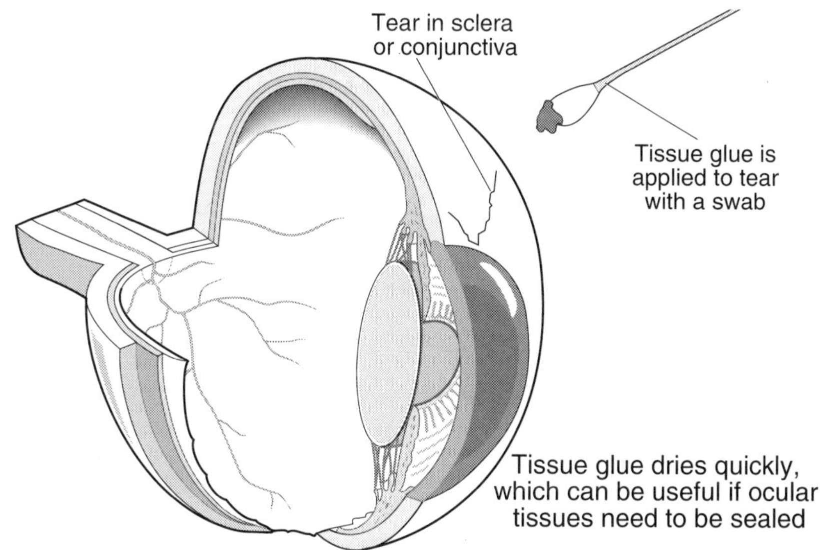

65400–65410* CPT CODES

CPT Description

65400 Excision of lesion, cornea (keratectomy, lamellar, partial), except pterygium

65410 Biopsy of cornea

Explanation

The physician removes the entire corneal lesion (e.g., 65400) using a blade and forceps or scleral scissors. The edges of the lesion are undermined following a superficial incision in the cornea. Sutures are not required. Antibiotic ointment and possibly a 24-hour pressure patch is applied. The lesion is superficial; the cornea is not perforated by the excision. Sometimes, only a portion of the lesion is removed for diagnostic purposes (e.g., 65410).

Comments

Caution: These codes are frequently – and erroneously – billed together. Remember that an excision reports the removal of an entire defect while a biopsy reports a sampling of the defect prior to its possible excision. When either the biopsy or excision specimen is taken to an outside laboratory for examination, report the conveyance of specimen with 99000. Also, note that 65410 is a starred procedure, and by definition reports only the surgical procedure performed. Any pre- or postoperative services performed in conjunction with 65410 are reported separately. This procedure is generally performed with a topical anesthetic rather than general anesthesia. Report the excision of a pterygium with 65420 or 65426. Report a diagnostic scraping of the cornea with 65320, and the destruction of a corneal lesion by cryotherapy, photocoagulation, or thermocauterization with 65450.

Commonly Associated ICD•9 Procedural Codes

11.22 Biopsy of cornea

11.49 Other removal or destruction of corneal lesion

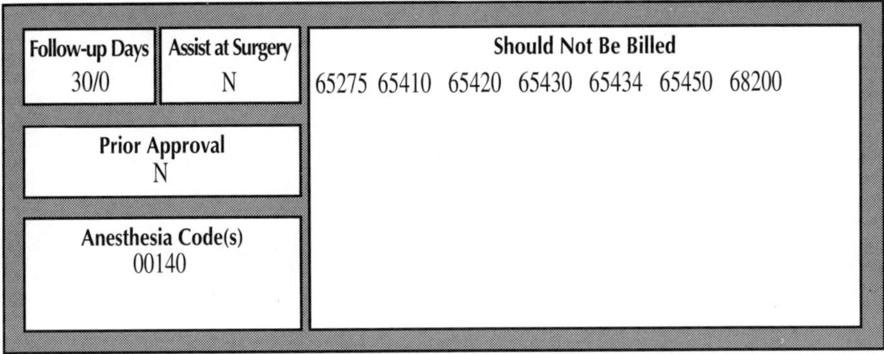

Follow-up Days	Assist at Surgery
30/0	N

Prior Approval
N

Anesthesia Code(s)
00140

Should Not Be Billed
65275 65410 65420 65430 65434 65450 68200

Commonly Associated ICD•9 Diagnostic Codes

190.4 Malignant neoplasm of cornea
224.4 Benign neoplasm of cornea
370.01 Marginal corneal ulcer
370.03 Central corneal ulcer
370.55 Corneal abscess
371.00 Corneal opacity, unspecified
371.10 Corneal deposit, unspecified
371.70 Corneal deformity, unspecified
371.70 Corneal deformity, unspecified
371.89 Other corneal disorders

Applicable HCPCS Level II Codes

A4550 Surgical tray

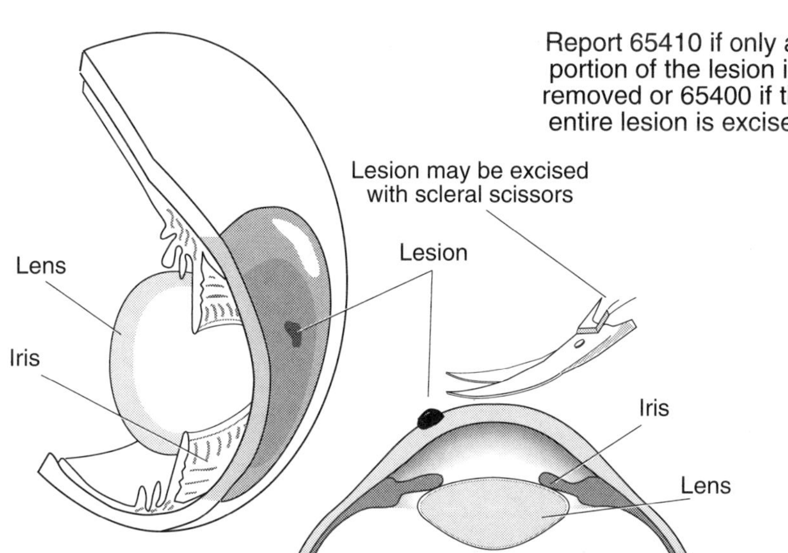

Lesion Excision

65420–65426 CPT CODES

CPT Description

65420 Excision or transposition of pterygium; without graft

65246 with graft

Explanation

A pterygium is a fleshy, wedge of the bulbar conjunctiva covering a portion of the medial cornea. The physician excises the pterygium with a blade and forceps or scleral scissors. The edges of the pterygium are undermined following a superficial incision in the clear cornea. Forceps retract the freed pterygium and it is excised as gentle pressure pulls it away from the corneal tissue and across the limbus and sclera. The physician applies sutures to the sclera and conjunctiva as needed. Often, no graft or tissue rearrangement is needed (e.g., 65420). However, the physician may transpose the pterygium with normal conjunctival tissue to move it out of the field of vision in what is sometimes called McReynold's operation, or may make a circumcorneal incision and use a conjunctival flap to repair the pterygium site (e.g., 65426). A topical antibiotic and a pressure patch may be applied in either procedure.

Comments

This procedure is generally performed with a subconjunctival injection or topical anesthetic rather than general anesthesia.

Commonly Associated ICD•9 Procedural Codes

11.31 Transposition of pterygium

11.32 Excision of pterygium with corneal graft

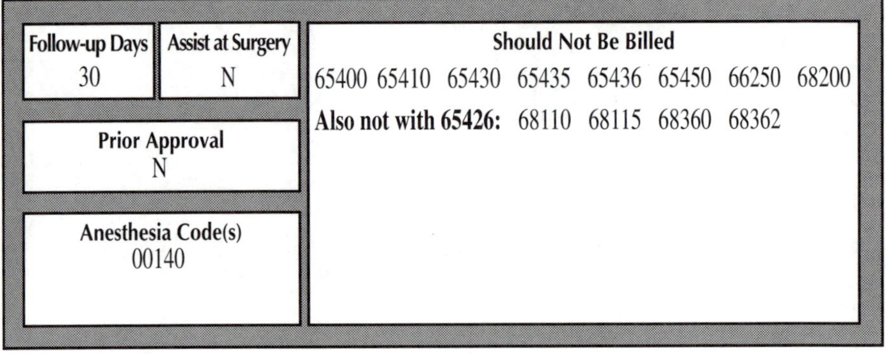

Follow-up Days
30

Assist at Surgery
N

Prior Approval
N

Anesthesia Code(s)
00140

Should Not Be Billed
65400 65410 65430 65435 65436 65450 66250 68200

Also not with 65426: 68110 68115 68360 68362

Commonly Associated ICD•9 Diagnostic Codes

372.40 Pterygium, unspecified
372.41 Peripheral pterygium, stationary
372.42 Peripheral pterygium, progressive
372.43 Central pterygium
372.44 Double pterygium
372.45 Recurrent pterygium
372.52 Pseudopterygium

Applicable HCPCS Level II Codes

A4305 Disposable drug delivery system, flow rate of 50 ml or greater per hour
A4306 Disposable drug delivery system, flow rate of 5 ml or less per hour
A4550 Surgical tray

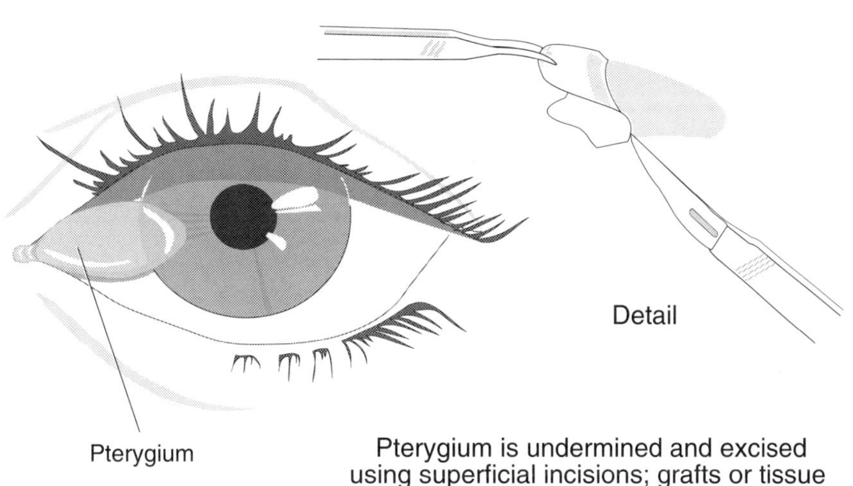

Pterygium Excision

65430* CPT CODE

CPT Description

Scraping of cornea, diagnostic, for smear and/or culture

Explanation

In the office, the physician scrapes the surface of the corneal defect with a spatula. The scrapings will be cultured to determine a diagnosis.

Comments

Report the conveyance of the specimen with 99000 if the specimen is taken to an outside laboratory. This procedure is generally performed with a subconjunctival injection or topical anesthetic rather than general anesthesia. This is a starred procedure, and by definition reports only the surgical procedure performed. Any pre- or postoperative services performed in conjunction with 65430 are reported separately. If tissue is cut from a corneal lesion, report a biopsy (65410) rather than a corneal scraping.

Commonly Associated ICD•9 Procedural Codes

11.21 Scraping of cornea for smear or culture

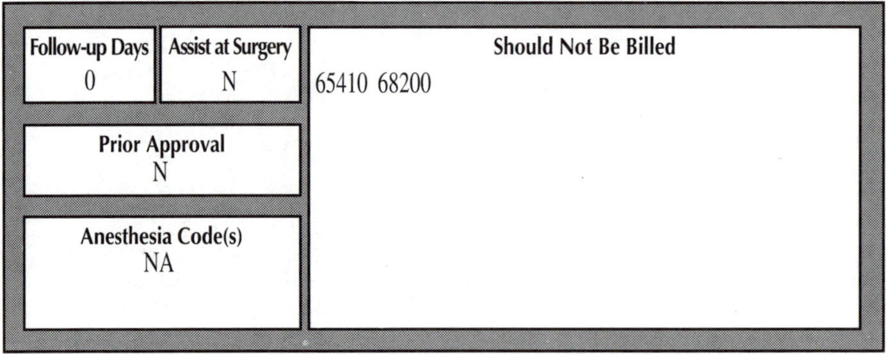

Follow-up Days	Assist at Surgery	Should Not Be Billed
0	N	65410 68200

Prior Approval
N

Anesthesia Code(s)
NA

Commonly Associated ICD•9 Diagnostic Codes

370.00 Corneal ulcer, unspecified
370.01 Marginal corneal ulcer
370.03 Central corneal ulcer
370.55 Corneal abscess
371.00 Corneal opacity, unspecified
371.10 Corneal deposit, unspecified
371.70 Corneal deformity, unspecified
371.89 Other corneal disorders

Applicable HCPCS Level II Codes

A4305 Disposable drug delivery system, flow rate of 50 ml or greater per hour
A4306 Disposable drug delivery system, flow rate of 5 ml or less per hour
A4550 Surgical tray

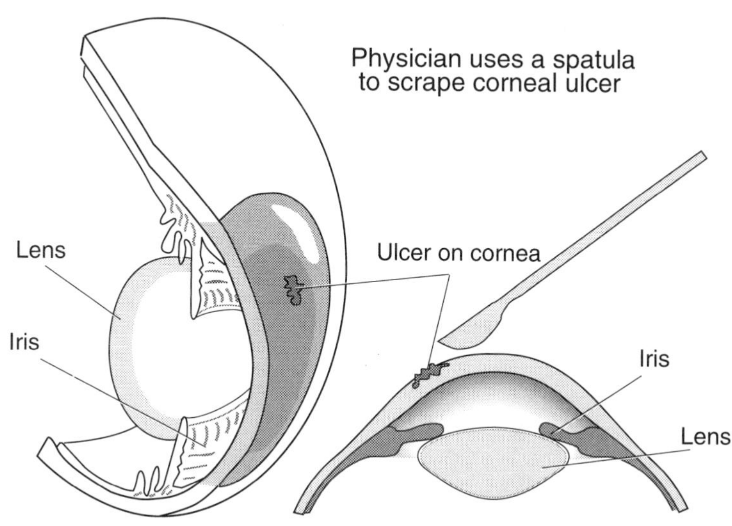

CPT Description

65435 Removal of corneal epithelium; with or without chemocauterization (abrasion, curettage)

65436 with application of chelating agent (eg, EDTA)

Explanation

In cases of corneal erosion or degeneration, the physician may attempt to stimulate new growth of the cornea's outermost layer by essentially "wounding" it. The physician removes the outermost layer of the cornea (epithelium) by scraping or cutting it with a spatula or curet (e.g., 65435). Chemical cauterization may then be applied. An alternative to cutting or scraping is the application by swab of EDTA (ethylenediaminetetraacetic acid), an acid that destroys the corneal epithelium. (e.g., 65436). In either case, an antibiotic ointment or pressure patch may be applied once the procedure is complete.

Comments

Note that 65435 is a starred procedure, and by definition reports only the surgical procedure performed. Any pre- or postoperative services performed in conjunction with 65435 are reported separately. This procedure is generally performed with a subconjunctival injection or a topical anesthetic rather than general anesthesia.

Commonly Associated ICD•9 Procedural Codes

11.41 Mechanical removal of corneal epithelium

11.49 Other removal or destruction of corneal lesion

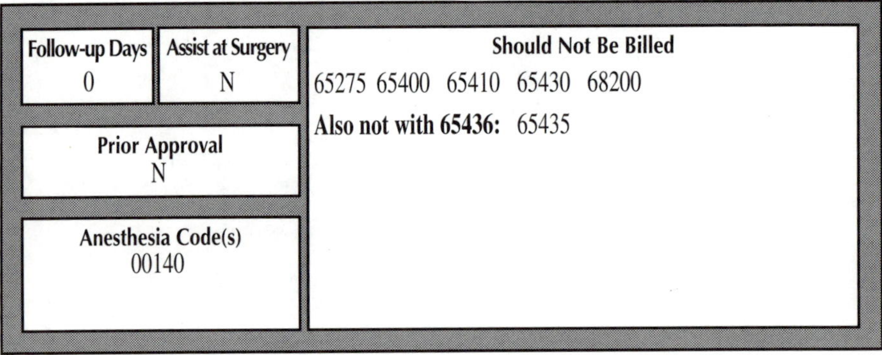

Follow-up Days	Assist at Surgery	Should Not Be Billed
0	N	65275 65400 65410 65430 68200
Prior Approval N		**Also not with 65436:** 65435
Anesthesia Code(s) 00140		

Commonly Associated ICD•9 Diagnostic Codes

364.1 Chronic iridocyclitis
371.43 Band-shaped keratopathy
371.44 Other calcerous degenerations of cornea

Applicable HCPCS Level II Codes

A4305 Disposable drug delivery system, flow rate of 50 ml or greater per hour
A4306 Disposable drug delivery system, flow rate of 5 ml or less per hour
A4550 Surgical tray

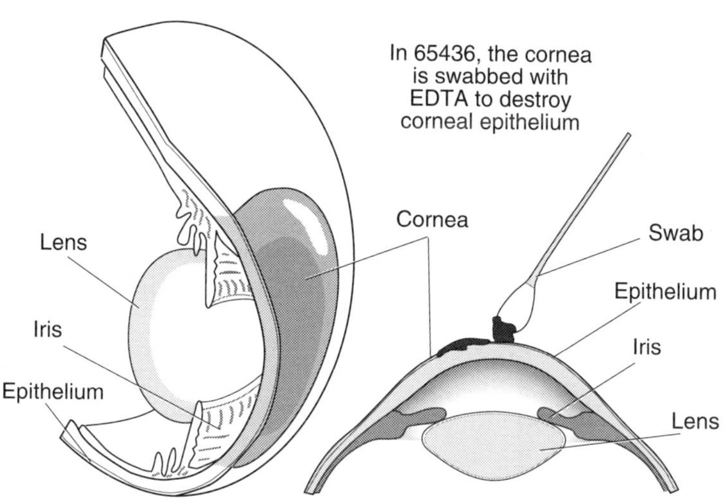

In 65435, the epithelium is removed with abrasion curettage

65450 CPT CODE

CPT Description

Destruction of lesion of cornea by cryotherapy, photocoagulation or thermocauterization

Explanation

The physician applies a freezing probe, a laser beam, or a heat probe directly to a corneal defect to destroy it. Freezing is the most common method used for this procedure. The physician then applies antibiotic ointment and sometimes, a pressure patch.

Comments

For excision of a corneal lesion, report 65400. This procedure is generally performed with a topical anesthetic or a subconjunctival injection rather than general anesthesia.

Commonly Associated ICD•9 Procedural Codes

11.42 Thermocauterization of corneal lesion
11.43 Cryotherapy of corneal lesion
11.49 Other removal or destruction of corneal lesion

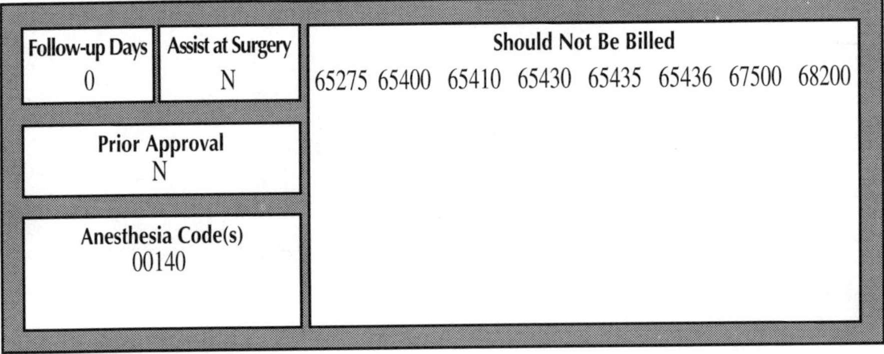

Follow-up Days	Assist at Surgery
0	N

Prior Approval
N

Anesthesia Code(s)
00140

Should Not Be Billed
65275 65400 65410 65430 65435 65436 67500 68200

Commonly Associated ICD•9 Diagnostic Codes

054.43 Herpes simplex disciform keratitis
090.3 Syphilitic interstitial keratitis
190.4 Malignant neoplasm of cornea
224.4 Benign neoplasm of cornea
370.00 Corneal ulcer, unspecified
370.55 Corneal abscess
371.70 Corneal deformity, unspecified
371.89 Other corneal disorders

Applicable HCPCS Level II Codes

A4305 Disposable drug delivery system, flow rate of 50 ml or greater per hour
A4306 Disposable drug delivery system, flow rate of 5 ml or less per hour
A4550 Surgical tray

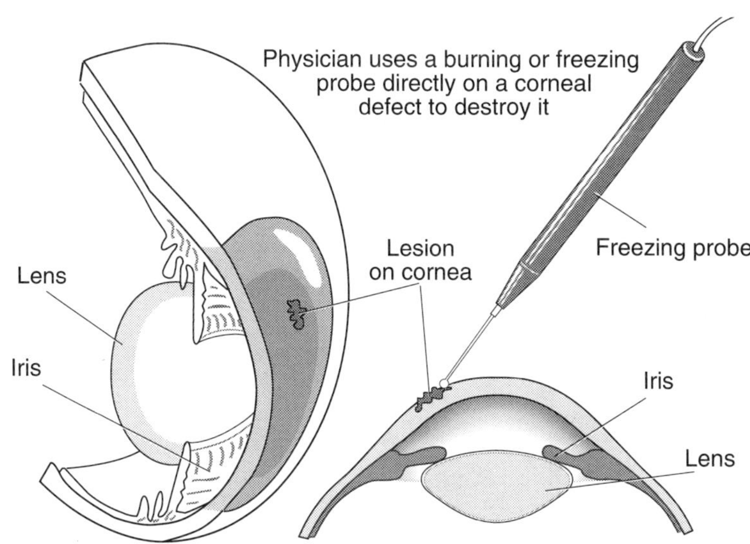

Corneal Lesion Destruction

65600 CPT CODE

CPT Description

Multiple punctures of anterior cornea (eg, for corneal erosion, tattoo)

Explanation

In cases of corneal erosion or degeneration, the physician may attempt to stimulate new growth of the cornea's outermost layer by essentially "wounding" it. The physician places a speculum in the eye and uses a fine needle to create hundreds of tiny pricks in the surface of the outermost layer of the cornea (the epithelium). A topical antibiotic and patch may be applied. This procedure is sometimes called a corneal "tattoo."

Comments

This procedure is generally performed with topical anesthetic rather than general anesthesia.

Commonly Associated ICD•9 Procedural Codes

11.91 Tattooing of cornea

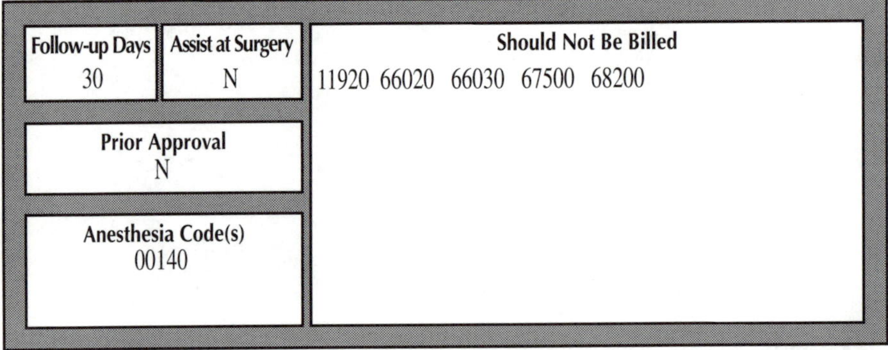

Follow-up Days	Assist at Surgery	Should Not Be Billed
30	N	11920 66020 66030 67500 68200

Prior Approval
N

Anesthesia Code(s)
00140

Commonly Associated ICD•9 Diagnostic Codes

054.43 Herpes simplex disciform keratitis
090.3 Syphilitic interstitial keratitis
224.4 Benign neoplasm of cornea
370.00 Corneal ulcer, unspecified
370.55 Corneal abscess
371.70 Corneal deformity, unspecified
371.89 Other corneal disorders

Applicable HCPCS Level II Codes

A4550 Surgical tray

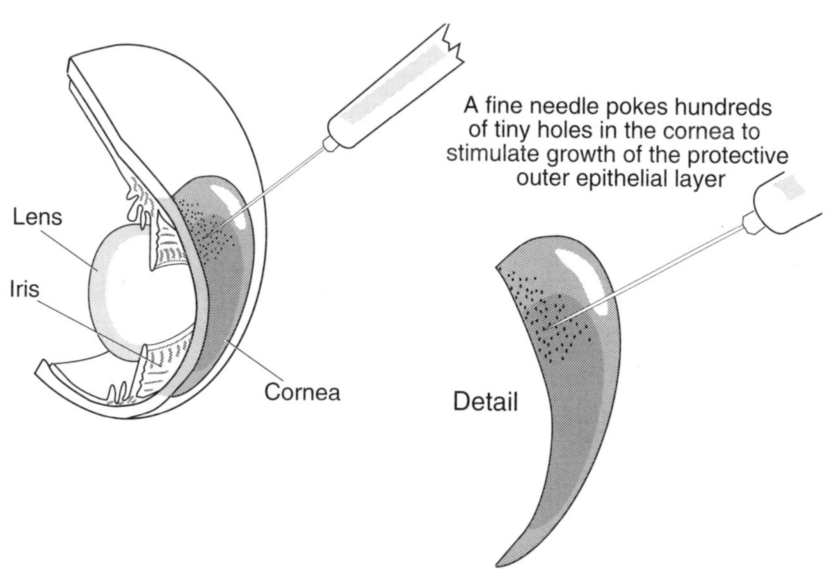

Multiple Punctures of Cornea

65710 CPT CODE

CPT Description

Keratoplasty (corneal transplant); lamellar

Explanation

"Lamellar" means thin layer, and refers to the outermost layers of the cornea. The physician measures the patient's cornea to select the size of trephine that will be used to excise corneal tissue. The physician punches a circular hole in the outermost layers of the cornea of a donor eye, using the trephine. The physician removes the round layer of corneal tissue, threads it with sutures, and sets it aside. The trephine is used to repeat this process in the cornea of the patient, removing the defective corneal tissue. The donor cornea is of similar diameter and thickness as the removed tissue. The donor cornea is positioned with the preplaced sutures, and then additional sutures secure it to the cornea. The physician may use a saline or air injection into the anterior chamber during the procedure. When the procedure is completed, the speculum is removed. Antibiotic ointment and a pressure patch may be applied.

Comments

All corneal transplant codes include the use of fresh or preserved grafts and the preparation by the physician of these materials. Do not use this code to report refractive keratoplasty procedures. For fitting of contact lens for treatment of disease, use 92070. This procedure is generally performed with a subconjunctival injection rather than general anesthesia. This code is also used to report the rotation of a patient's own lamellar corneal tissue in an uncommon procedure where the patient's corneal tissue is excised, rotated and reattached to move a corneal defect out of the visual field.

Commonly Associated ICD•9 Procedural Codes

11.61 Lamellar keratoplasty with autograft
11.62 Other lamellar keratoplasty

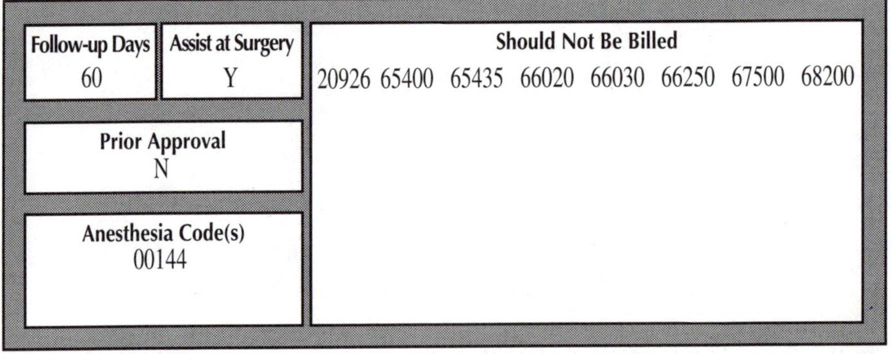

Follow-up Days	Assist at Surgery	Should Not Be Billed
60	Y	20926 65400 65435 66020 66030 66250 67500 68200

Prior Approval
N

Anesthesia Code(s)
00144

Commonly Associated ICD•9 Diagnostic Codes

371.01 Minor opacity of cornea
371.02 Peripheral opacity of cornea
371.03 Central opacity of cornea
371.11 Anterior corneal pigmentations
371.12 Stromal corneal pigmentations
371.13 Posterior corneal pigmentations
371.30 Corneal membrane change, unspecified
371.41 Senile corneal changes

Applicable HCPCS Level II Codes

A4305 Disposable drug delivery system, flow rate of 50 ml or greater per hour
A4306 Disposable drug delivery system, flow rate of 5 ml or less per hour
A4550 Surgical tray
V2785 Processing, preserving and transporting corneal tissue

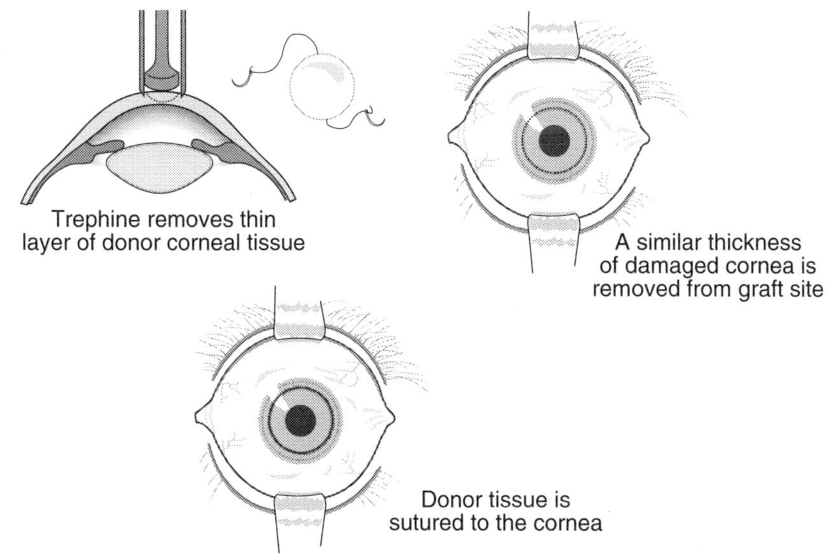

65730–65755 CPT CODES

CPT Description

65730 Keratoplasty (corneal transplant); penetrating (except in aphakia)

65750 penetrating (in aphakia)

65755 penetrating (in pseudophakia)

Explanation

Penetrating refers to the thickness of the donor cornea, indicating it is full thickness. The physician measures the patient's cornea to select the size of trephine that will be used to excise corneal tissue. The physician punches a circular hole in the cornea of the donor eye using the trephine. The physician removes the disk of corneal tissue, threads it with preplaced sutures, and sets it aside. In aphakic patients, vitreous and/or aqueous may be withdrawn from the eye before the cornea is removed. A metal ring may be sutured to the sclera of an aphakic patient to stabilize the operative field. The defective cornea of the patient is removed with the trephine. The donor cornea is positioned with sutures, and then additional sutures secure it to the cornea. The physician may use a saline or air injection to restore proper intraocular pressure.

Comments

The difference in these three codes is the lens status of the patient. 65730 is for those who still have a natural lens: these patients are phakic – with lens. 65750 is for those who have had cataract surgery: these patients are aphakic – without lens. 65755 is for those who have an artificial intraocular lens: these patients are pseudoaphakic – without natural lens. This procedure is generally performed with a subconjunctival or retrobulbar injection rather than general anesthesia. These codes also are used to report the rotation of a patient's own corneal tissue in an uncommon procedure where the corneal tissue is excised, rotated and reattached to move a corneal defect out of the visual field.

Commonly Associated ICD•9 Procedural Codes

11.63 Penetrating keratoplasty with autograft

11.64 Other penetrating keratoplasty

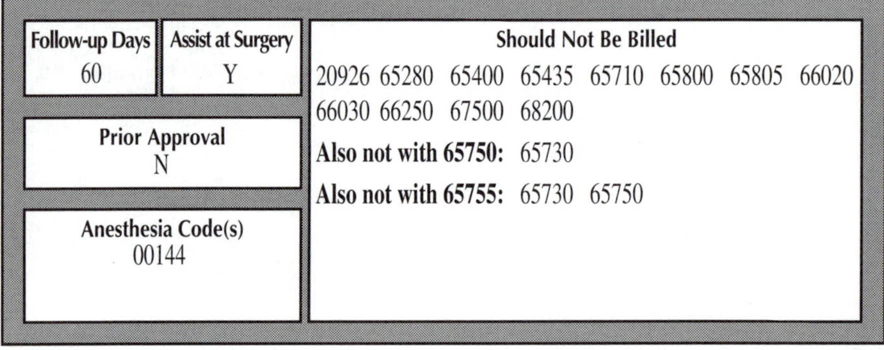

Follow-up Days	Assist at Surgery
60	Y

Prior Approval
N

Anesthesia Code(s)
00144

Should Not Be Billed

20926 65280 65400 65435 65710 65800 65805 66020 66030 66250 67500 68200

Also not with 65750: 65730

Also not with 65755: 65730 65750

Commonly Associated ICD•9 Diagnostic Codes

264.6 Vitamin A deficiency with xerophthalmic scars of cornea
370.63 Deep vascularization of cornea
371.02 Peripheral opacity of cornea
371.03 Central opacity of cornea
371.04 Adherent leucoma
371.20 Corneal edema, unspecified
371.23 Bullous keratopathy
371.31 Folds and rupture of Bowman's membrane
371.46 Nodular degeneration of cornea
371.53 Granular corneal dystrophy
371.6 Keratoconus
743.42 Congenital corneal opacities, interfering with vision
871.0 Ocular laceration without prolapse of intraocular tissue
871.1 Ocular laceration with prolapse or exposure of intraocular tissue
871.9 Unspecified open wound of eyeball

Also for 65750:
379.31 Aphakia

Applicable HCPCS Level II Codes

A4305 Disposable drug delivery system, flow rate of 50 ml or greater per hour
A4306 Disposable drug delivery system, flow rate of 5 ml or less per hour
A4550 Surgical tray
V2785 Processing, preserving and transporting corneal tissue

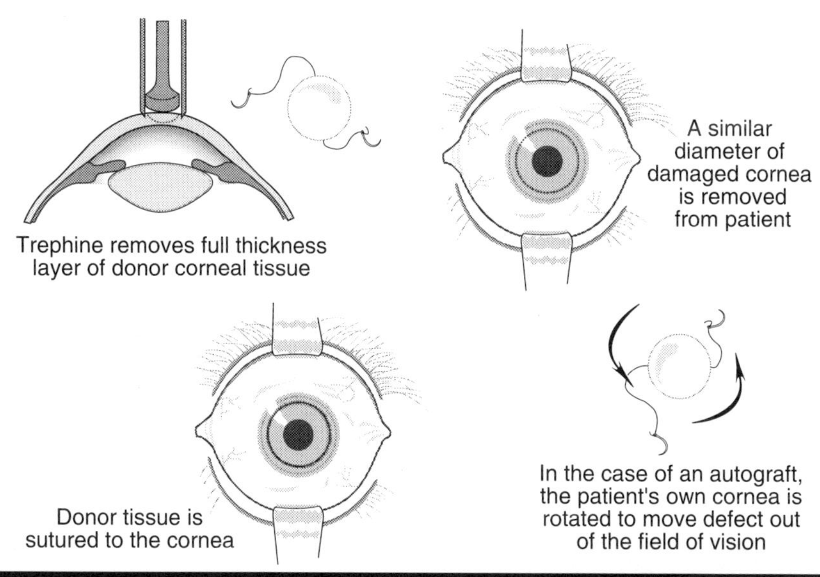

KERATOPLASTY

65760 CPT CODE

CPT Description

Keratomileusis

Explanation

The cornea is one of several structures in the eye that contributes to refraction. Altering the shape of the cornea therefore alters visual acuity. The physician retracts the patient's eyelids with an ocular speculum. Using a planing device, the physician removes a partial-thickness central portion of the patient's cornea, freezes it and then reshapes it on an electronic lathe. The revised cornea is positioned and secured with sutures. This is done to correct optical error. The physician may use a saline or air injection into the anterior chamber during the procedure. The speculum is removed. Antibiotic ointment and a pressure patch may be applied.

Comments

Code with caution: This procedure, performed to correct high degrees of myopia, has largely been replaced by the anterior lamellar keretoplasty (ALK), which should be reported with 66999 *Unlisted procedure, anterior chamber of eye.* A cover letter should accompany the claim.

Commonly Associated ICD•9 Procedural Codes

11.71 Keratomeleusis

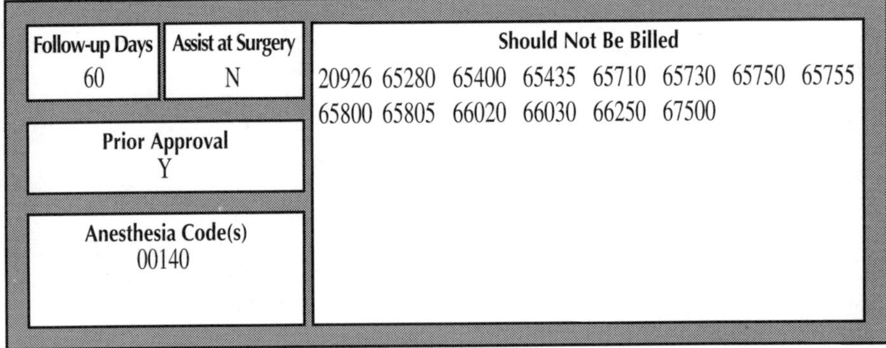

Follow-up Days	Assist at Surgery
60	N

Prior Approval
Y

Anesthesia Code(s)
00140

Should Not Be Billed
20926 65280 65400 65435 65710 65730 65750 65755
65800 65805 66020 66030 66250 67500

Commonly Associated ICD•9 Diagnostic Codes

367.89 Other disorders of refraction and accommodation
367.9 Unspecified disorder of refraction and accommodation
371.61 Keratoconus, stable condition
371.62 Keratoconus, acute hydrops
371.70 Corneal deformity, unspecified

Applicable HCPCS Level II Codes

A4305 Disposable drug delivery system, flow rate of 50 ml or greater per hour
A4306 Disposable drug delivery system, flow rate of 5 ml or less per hour
A4550 Surgical tray

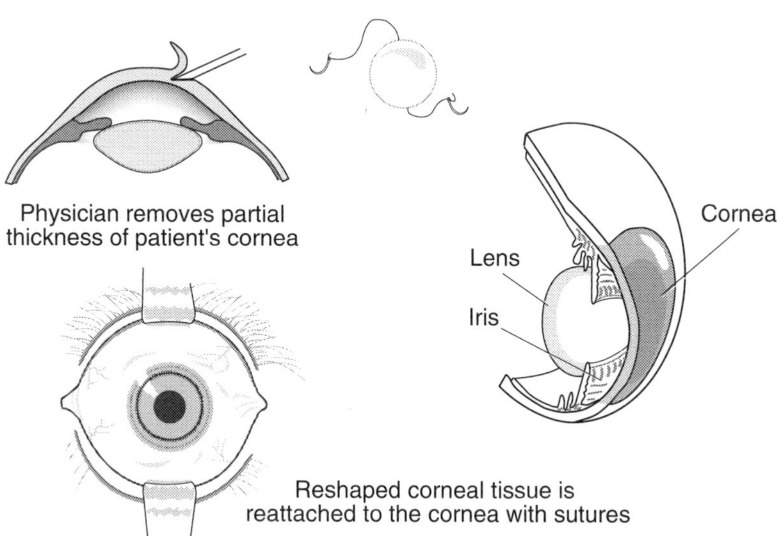

65765 CPT CODE

CPT Description

Keratophakia

Explanation

The cornea is one of several structures in the eye that contributes to refraction. Altering the shape of the cornea therefore alters visual acuity. The physician retracts the patient's eyelids with an ocular speculum, then measures the patient's cornea to select the size of trephine that will be used to excise corneal tissue. The physician punches a circular hole in the cornea of the donor eye using the trephine. The physician removes the disk of corneal tissue and sets it aside. An incision is made at the juncture of the cornea and the sclera (the limbus) and the patient's cornea is separated into two layers. The physician inserts the donor cornea between layers of the recipient's cornea. The resulting change in the corneal curvature alters the refractive properties of the cornea to correct the preexisting refractive error. The speculum is removed. Antibiotic ointment and a pressure patch may be applied.

Comments

Because the correction of a refractive error is usually not done out of medical necessity, patients are usually responsible for all charges. This procedure is generally performed with a subconjunctival or retrobulbar injection rather than general anesthesia.

Commonly Associated ICD•9 Procedural Codes

11.72 Keratophakia

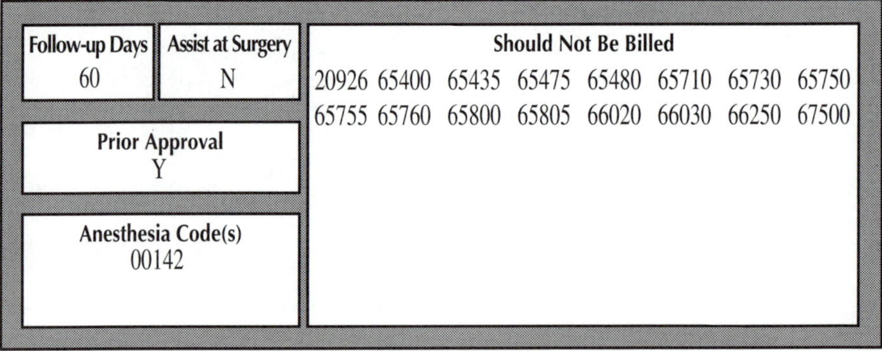

Follow-up Days	Assist at Surgery
60	N

Prior Approval
Y

Anesthesia Code(s)
00142

Should Not Be Billed

20926 65400 65435 65475 65480 65710 65730 65750
65755 65760 65800 65805 66020 66030 66250 67500

Commonly Associated ICD•9 Diagnostic Codes

367.1 Myopia
367.89 Other disorders of refraction and accommodation
367.9 Unspecified disorder of refraction and accommodation

Applicable HCPCS Level II Codes

A4305 Disposable drug delivery system, flow rate of 50 ml or greater per hour
A4306 Disposable drug delivery system, flow rate of 5 ml or less per hour
A4550 Surgical tray
V2785 Processing, preserving and transporting corneal tissue

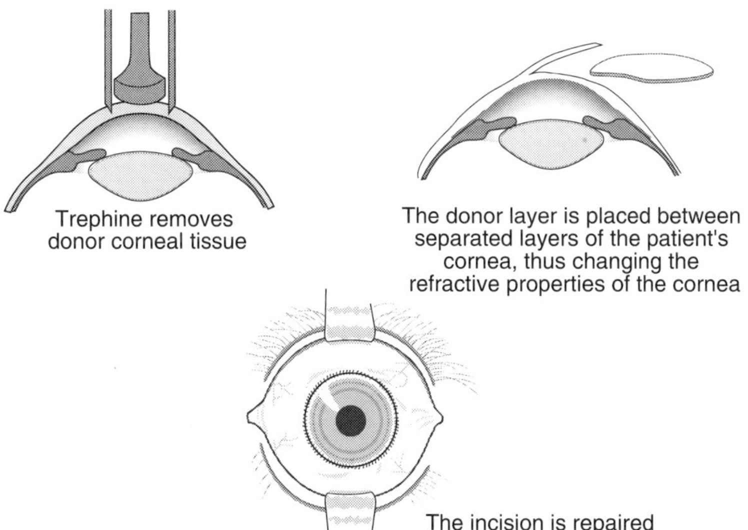

65767 CPT CODE

CPT Description

Epikeratoplasty

Explanation

The cornea is one of several structures in the eye that contributes to refraction. Altering the shape of the cornea therefore alters visual acuity. The physician retracts the patient's eyelids with an ocular speculum, then measures the patient's cornea to select the size of trephine that will be used to excise corneal tissue. The physician punches a circular hole in the cornea of the donor eye using the trephine. The physician removes the disk of corneal tissue and sets it aside. On a lathe, the physician shapes a lens made of two layers from a donor cornea, the stroma and Bowman's membrane. The physician sutures this donor cornea to the surface of the patient's cornea. The resulting change in the corneal curvature alters the refractive properties of the cornea to correct the preexisting refractive error. The speculum is removed. Antibiotic ointment and a pressure patch may be applied.

Comments

Because the correction of a refractive error is usually not done out of medical necessity, patients are generally responsible for all charges. However, in cases where patients are aphakic (without lens) and lens implantation is contraindicated, reimbursement is considered if a cover letter accompanies the claim. This procedure is generally performed with a subconjunctival or retrobulbar injection rather than general anesthesia.

Commonly Associated ICD•9 Procedural Codes

11.76 Epikeratophakia

11.79 Other reconstructive surgery on cornea

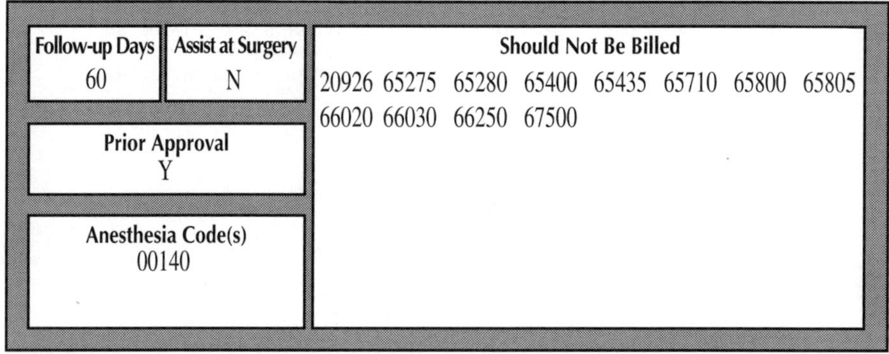

Follow-up Days	Assist at Surgery	Should Not Be Billed
60	N	20926 65275 65280 65400 65435 65710 65800 65805 66020 66030 66250 67500
Prior Approval Y		
Anesthesia Code(s) 00140		

Commonly Associated ICD•9 Diagnostic Codes

367.1 Myopia
367.89 Other disorders of refraction and accommodation
367.9 Unspecified disorder of refraction and accommodation
371.61 Keratoconus, stable condition
379.31 Aphakia
743.35 Congenital aphakia
996.53 Mechanical complication of ocular lens prosthesis

Applicable HCPCS Level II Codes

A4305 Disposable drug delivery system, flow rate of 50 ml or greater per hour
A4306 Disposable drug delivery system, flow rate of 5 ml or less per hour
A4550 Surgical tray
V2785 Processing, preserving and transporting corneal tissue

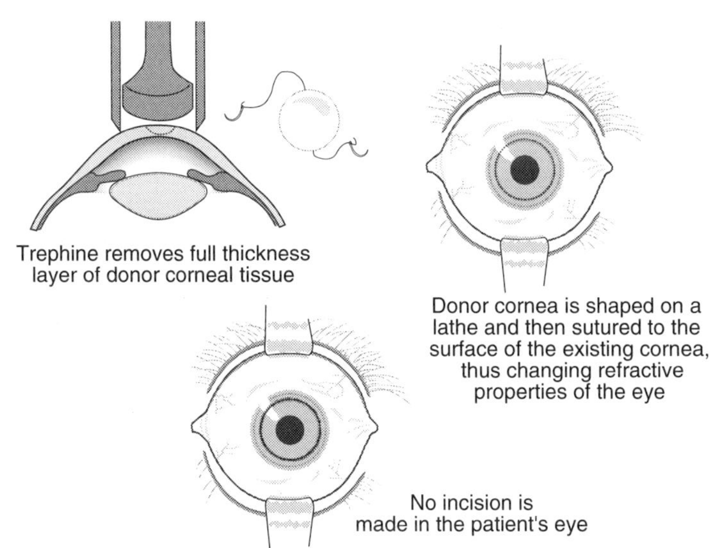

65770 CPT CODE

CPT Description

Keratoprosthesis

Explanation

The physician creates a new anterior chamber with a plastic optical implant that replaces a severely damaged cornea that cannot be repaired. Sometimes the corneal prosthesis is sutured to the sclera; other times, extensive damage to the eye requires the implant be sutured to the closed and incised eyelid.

Comments

Code with caution; this procedure is rarely used. Include a cover letter and a copy of the operative report. This procedure is generally performed with a retrobulbar injection rather than general anesthesia.

Commonly Associated ICD•9 Procedural Codes

11.73 Keratoprosthesis

Follow-up Days	Assist at Surgery
60	N

Prior Approval
Y

Anesthesia Code(s)
00144

Should Not Be Billed

12051	12052	12053	12054	12055	13150	13151	13152
65270	65272	65273	65275	65280	65285	65286	65290
65730	65750	65755	65810	65815	65930	66020	66030
66250	67005	67015	67025	67028	67875	67880	67882
68110	68115	68130	68135				

Commonly Associated ICD•9 Diagnostic Codes

076.1 Trachoma, active stage
694.61 Benign mucous membrane pemphigoid with ocular involvement
695.1 Erythema multiforme
871.0 Ocular laceration without prolapse of intraocular tissue
871.2 Rupture of eye with partial loss of intraocular tissue
891.9 Other burn of cornea and conjunctival sac
940.2 Alkaline chemical burn of cornea and conjunctival sac
940.3 Acid chemical burn of cornea and conjunctival sac
940.4 Other burn of cornea and conjunctival sac
996.51 Mechanical complication of corneal graft

Applicable HCPCS Level II Codes

A4305 Disposable drug delivery system, flow rate of 50 ml or greater per hour
A4306 Disposable drug delivery system, flow rate of 5 ml or less per hour
A4550 Surgical tray
V2599 Contact lens, other type

The procedure tries to re-create the anterior chamber of a damaged eye

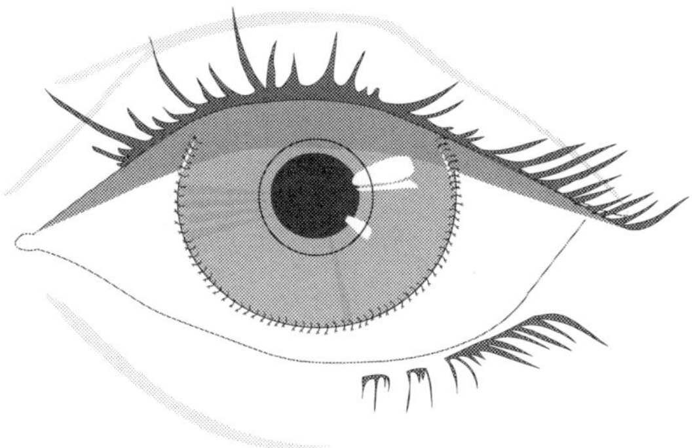

Sometimes the corneal prosthesis is sutured to the sclera in this rarely performed surgery

65771 CPT CODE

CPT Description

Radial keratotomy

Explanation

The cornea is one of several structures in the eye that contributes to refraction. Altering the shape of the cornea therefore alters visual acuity. The physician retracts the patient's eyelids with an ocular speculum, then measures the patient's cornea. The physician places multiple nonpenetrating cuts in the cornea in a bicycle spoke on the patient's corneal to reduce myopia, or a variety of peripheral cornea tangential cuts for astigmatic correction. There are two basic surgical approaches: Russian, in which the incisions are made from the edges to the center of the cornea; and American, in which the incisions are made from the center to the periphery. The number and length of the incisions depends upon the patient's age and degree of myopia. The resulting change in the corneal curvature alters the refractive properties of the cornea to correct the preexisting refractive error. The speculum is removed. Antibiotic ointment and a pressure patch may be applied.

Comments

Because the correction of a refractive error is usually not done out of medical necessity, patients are generally responsible for all charges. However, some insurance companies will cover this procedure if preauthorized. This procedure is generally performed with a subconjunctival or retrobulbar injection rather than general anesthesia.

Commonly Associated ICD•9 Procedural Codes

11.75 Radial keratotomy

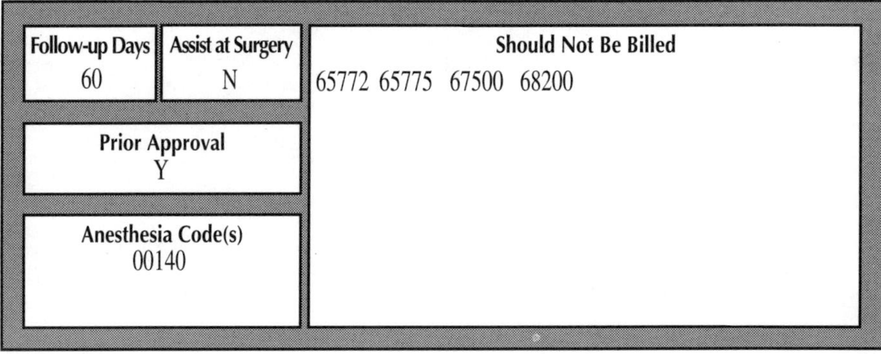

Follow-up Days	Assist at Surgery	Should Not Be Billed
60	N	65772 65775 67500 68200

Prior Approval
Y

Anesthesia Code(s)
00140

Commonly Associated ICD•9 Diagnostic Codes

367.1 Myopia

Applicable HCPCS Level II Codes

A4305 Disposable drug delivery system, flow rate of 50 ml or greater per hour
A4306 Disposable drug delivery system, flow rate of 5 ml or less per hour
A4550 Surgical tray

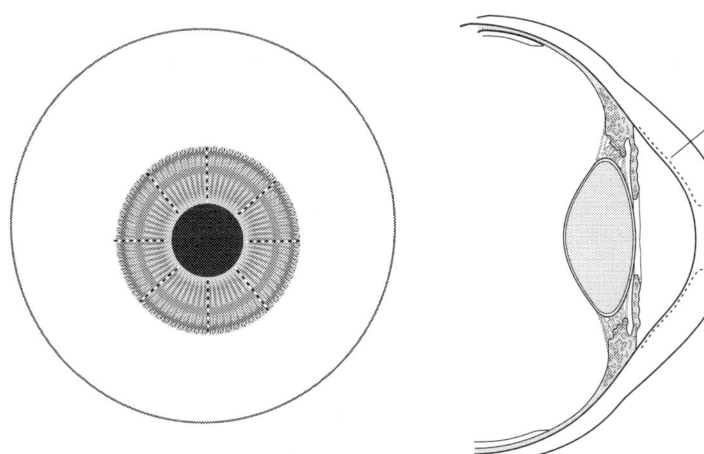

Radial incisions extend from optical zone to limbus

Cross-section view

RADIAL KERATOTOMY

CPT Description

65772 Corneal relaxing incision for correction of surgically induced astigmatism

65775 Corneal wedge resection for correction of surgically induced astigmatism

Explanation

The cornea is one of several structures in the eye that contributes to refraction. Altering the shape of the cornea therefore alters visual acuity. When a previous surgery (e.g., for insertion of an intraocular lens or a corneal procedure) results in astigmatism, the physician at a later date returns the patient to the operating room to correct the problem.The physician retracts the patient's eyelids with an ocular speculum. In corneal relaxing (65772), an "X" cut is made on the cornea to repair the error. Slices along the "X" are removed and its edges are sutured. In the corneal wedge resection (65775), a wedge is cut from the cornea and the edges sutured. The resulting change in the corneal curvature alters the refractive properties of the cornea to correct the preexisting refractive error. The speculum is removed. Antibiotic ointment and a pressure patch may be applied.

Comments

The corneal relaxing procedure is rarely done anymore; most physicians prefer the wedge procedure. Medicare will only pay for one procedure per eye for the life of the patient. Some payers require the repair to be performed within a certain time frame (e.g., within one year of the original surgery). This procedure is generally performed with a subconjunctival or retrobulbar injection rather than general anesthesia.

Commonly Associated ICD•9 Procedural Codes

11.79 Other reconstructive surgery on cornea

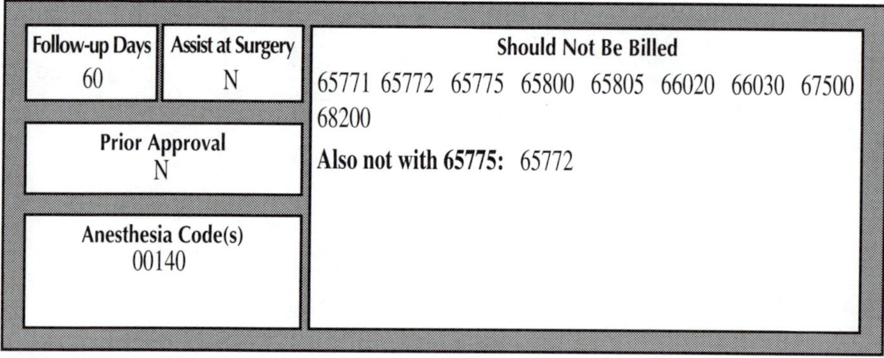

Follow-up Days	Assist at Surgery	Should Not Be Billed
60	N	65771 65772 65775 65800 65805 66020 66030 67500 68200
Prior Approval		**Also not with 65775:** 65772
N		
Anesthesia Code(s)		
00140		

Commonly Associated ICD•9 Diagnostic Codes

367.21 Regular astigmatism

367.22 Irregular astigmatism

E878.4 Other restorative surgery causing abnormal patient reaction, or later complication, without mention of misadventure at time of operation

Applicable HCPCS Level II Codes

A4305 Disposable drug delivery system, flow rate of 50 ml or greater per hour

A4306 Disposable drug delivery system, flow rate of 5 ml or less per hour

A4550 Surgical tray

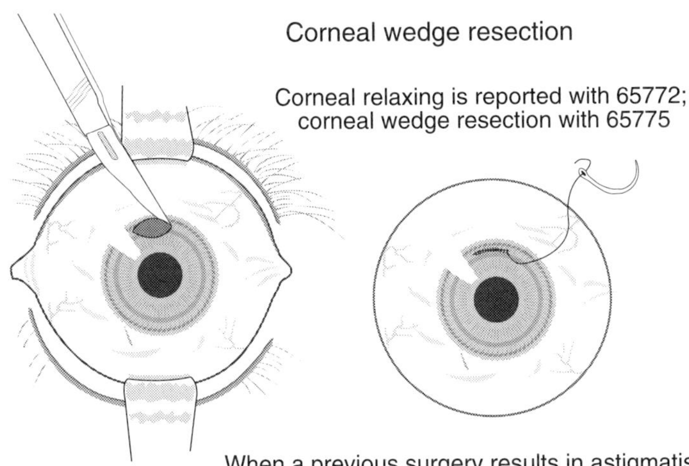

65800*–65805* CPT CODES

CPT Description

65800 Paracentesis of anterior chamber of eye (separate procedure); with diagnostic aspiration of aqueous

65805 with therapeutic release of aqueous

Explanation

Though constantly flushed and renewed, the overall pressure of aqueous is constant in a healthy eye's anterior chamber. Too little or too much fluid can cause permanent damage. The physician aspirates aqueous from between the iris and the cornea (the anterior chamber) with a needle in what is typically called an "anterior chamber tap." The needle usually enters the anterior chamber through the corneal-scleral juncture (the limbus). In some cases, the removal of the fluid is diagnostic (e.g., 65800). The physician may inject air to normalize eye pressure after fluid has been removed. If ocular pressure is high, a therapeutic removal of aqueous may be performed (e.g., 65805).

Comments

Code 65800 reports paracentesis that is usually a component of larger, more complicated procedure. As such, it is not separately reported. However, if paracentesis alone is performed, use 65800 to report the separate procedure. Also note that 65800 and 65805 are starred codes, and as such, report only the procedure. Any pre- or postoperative service can be reported separately. This procedure is generally performed with a topical anesthetic rather than general anesthesia. For injection into the anterior chamber, see 66020 and 66030.

Commonly Associated ICD•9 Procedural Codes

12.21 Diagnostic aspiration of anterior chamber of eye

12.91 Therapeutic evacuation of anterior chamber

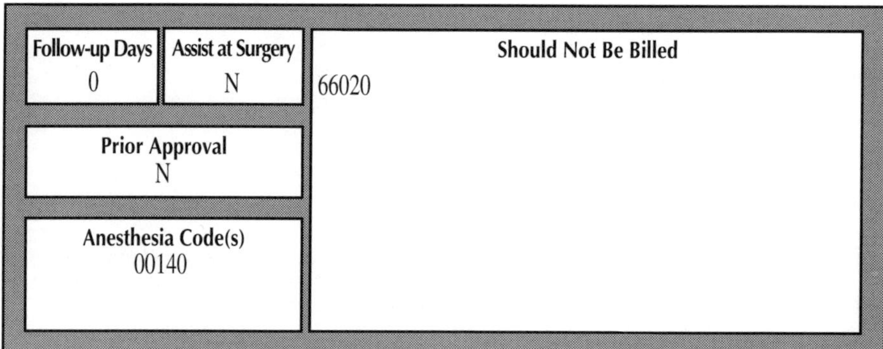

Follow-up Days	Assist at Surgery	Should Not Be Billed
0	N	66020
Prior Approval		
N		
Anesthesia Code(s)		
00140		

Commonly Associated ICD•9 Diagnostic Codes

For 65800:

364.05 Hypopyon

For 65805

365.22 Acute angle-closure glaucoma
365.59 Glaucoma associated with other lens disorders
365.62 Glaucoma associated with ocular inflammations
365.64 Glaucoma associated with tumors or cysts
365.65 Glaucoma associated with ocular trauma

Applicable HCPCS Level II Codes

A4305 Disposable drug delivery system, flow rate of 50 ml or greater per hour
A4306 Disposable drug delivery system, flow rate of 5 ml or less per hour
A4550 Surgical tray

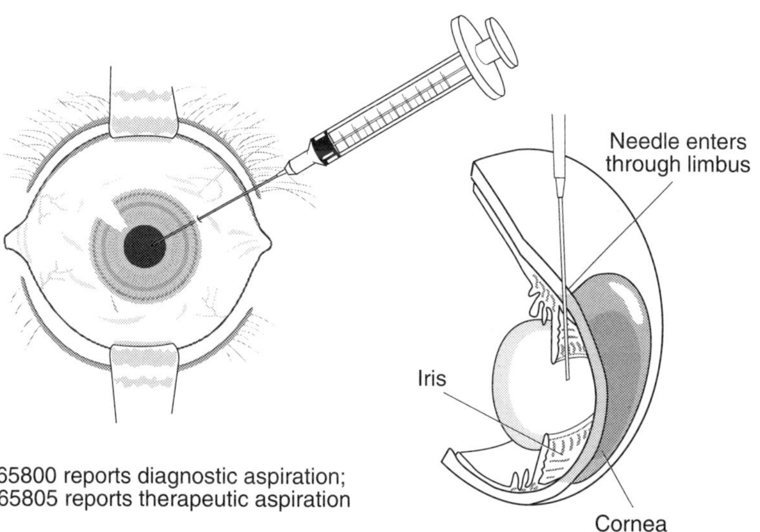

65800 reports diagnostic aspiration;
65805 reports therapeutic aspiration

65810 CPT CODE

CPT Description

Paracentesis of anterior chamber of eye (separate procedure); with removal of vitreous and/or discission of anterior hyaloid membrane, with or without air injection

Explanation

The physician aspirates the gel-like vitreous that has pushed forward into the space between the iris and the cornea (the anterior chamber). Using a needle that enters the eye through the corneal-scleral juncture (the limbus), the prolapsed vitreous is removed. A laser might be used to destroy part of the membrane between the lens and the vitreous (the anterior hyaloid membrane). The physician may inject air to normalize eye pressure after fluid has been removed.

Comments

This code reports paracentesis that is usually a component of a larger, more complicated procedure. As such, it is not separately reported. However, if paracentesis is performed solely with the removal of vitreous and/or discission of anterior hyaloid membrane, use 65810 to report the separate procedure. This procedure is generally performed with a subconjunctival injection rather than general anesthesia.

Commonly Associated ICD•9 Procedural Codes

14.71 Removal of vitreous, anterior approach

12.91 Therapeutic evacuation of anterior chamber

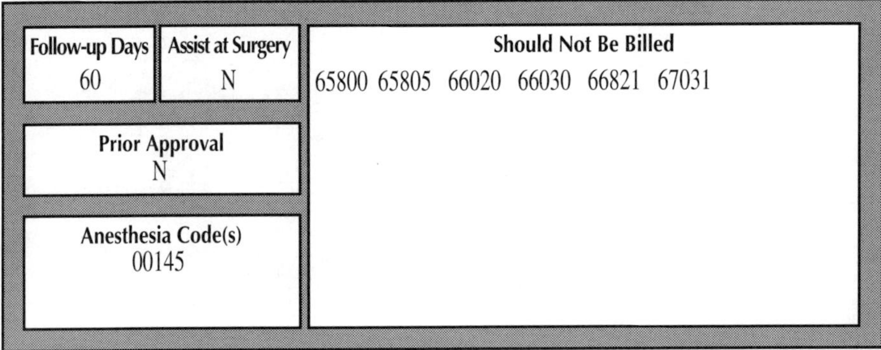

Follow-up Days	Assist at Surgery	Should Not Be Billed
60	N	65800 65805 66020 66030 66821 67031

Prior Approval
N

Anesthesia Code(s)
00145

Commonly Associated ICD•9 Diagnostic Codes

364.74 Adhesions and disruptions of pupillary membranes
365.61 Glaucoma associated with pupillary block
379.26 Vitreous prolapse

Applicable HCPCS Level II Codes

A4305 Disposable drug delivery system, flow rate of 50 ml or greater per hour
A4306 Disposable drug delivery system, flow rate of 5 ml or less per hour
A4550 Surgical tray

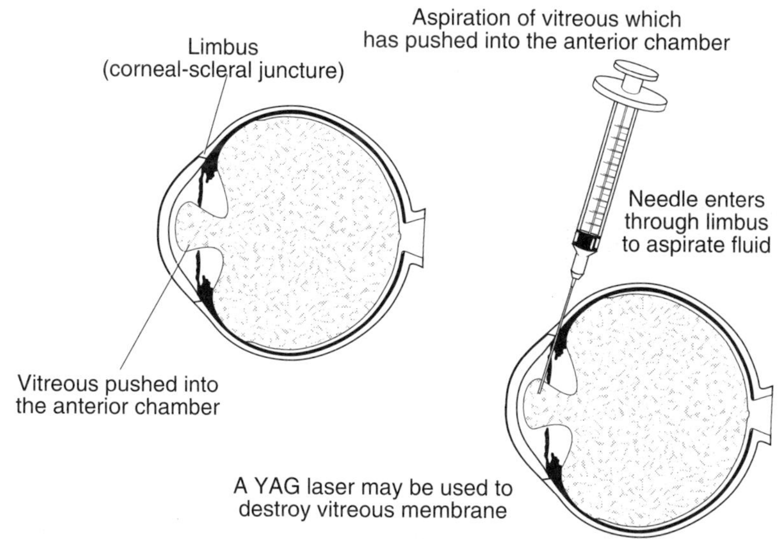

PARACENTESIS

65815 CPT CODE

CPT Description

Paracentesis of anterior chamber of eye (separate procedure); with removal of blood, with or without irrigation and/or air injection

Explanation

Blood in the anterior chamber can coagulate and block the flow of aqueous. It can also cause cornea staining. The physician aspirates blood from between the iris and the cornea (the anterior chamber) with a needle that enters the eye through the corneal-scleral juncture (the limbus). In some cases, the physician may inject saline to flush the blood and make its removal easier. The physician may inject air to normalize eye pressure after fluid has been removed.

Comments

This code reports paracentesis that is usually a component of a larger, more complicated procedure. As such, it is not reported separately. However, if paracentesis is performed solely with the removal of blood from the anterior chamber, use 65810 to report the separate procedure. Note that 65815 reports the aspiration of blood, and should not be confused with 65930, which reports aspiration of a blood clot. This procedure is generally performed with a subconjunctival injection rather than general anesthesia.

Commonly Associated ICD•9 Procedural Codes

12.91 Therapeutic evacuation of anterior chamber

Follow-up Days	Assist at Surgery
30	N

Prior Approval
N

Anesthesia Code(s)
00140

Should Not Be Billed
65800 65805 65810 65930 66020 66030 67500 68500

Commonly Associated ICD•9 Diagnostic Codes

364.41 Hyphema of iris and ciliary body
365.64 Glaucoma associated with tumors or cysts

Applicable HCPCS Level II Codes

A4305 Disposable drug delivery system, flow rate of 50 ml or greater per hour
A4306 Disposable drug delivery system, flow rate of 5 ml or less per hour
A4550 Surgical tray

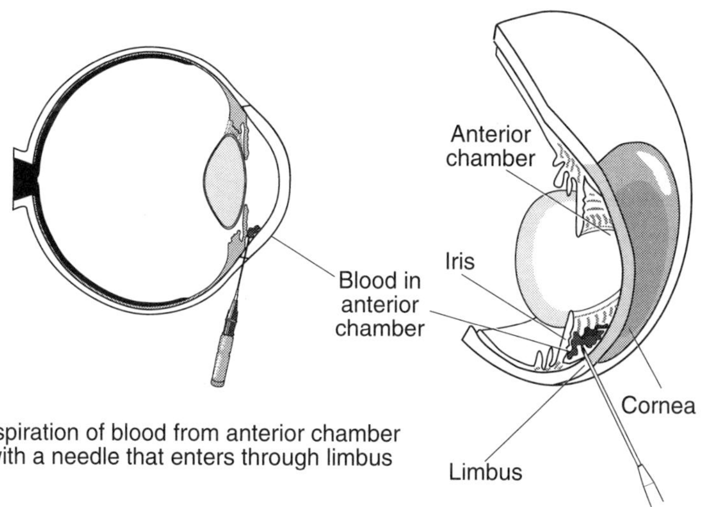

Aspiration of blood from anterior chamber with a needle that enters through limbus

65820 CPT CODE

CPT Description

Goniotomy

Explanation

Though constantly flushed and renewed, the overall pressure of aqueous is constant in a healthy eye's anterior chamber. Too little or too much fluid can cause permanent damage. To improve drainage of fluids in the eye, the physician enters the anterior chamber through an incision in the scleral-corneal juncture (the limbus) and cuts with a gonioknife. The blade passes across the anterior to the opposite limbus and a sweep is made to open the angle of the ring of meshlike tissue at the iris-scleral junction (the trabecular meshwork) of the opposite portion of the eye. De Vincentiis operation and Barkan's operation are both goniotomy procedures.

Comments

This procedure requires a clear cornea for adequate visualization. No tissue is removed. If the trabecular meshwork is approached from outside the eye instead of from across the anterior segment, report 65850. A gonioscopy is performed for this procedure and can be reported separately with 92020. This procedure is generally performed with a subconjunctival or retrobulbar injection rather than general anesthesia.

Commonly Associated ICD•9 Procedural Codes

12.52 Goniotomy without goniopuncture

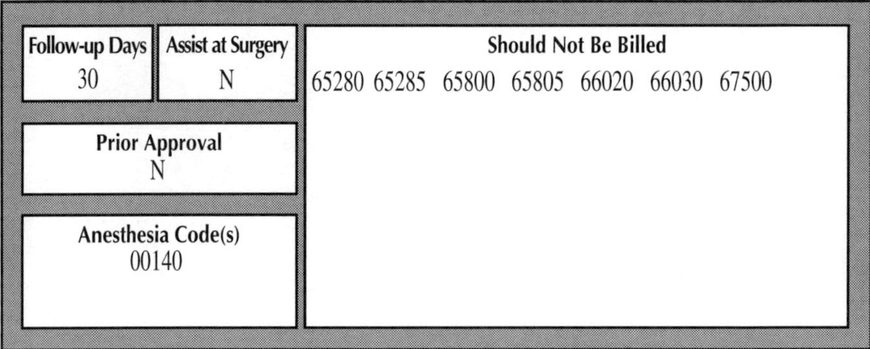

Follow-up Days	Assist at Surgery	Should Not Be Billed
30	N	65280 65285 65800 65805 66020 66030 67500

Prior Approval
N

Anesthesia Code(s)
00140

Commonly Associated ICD•9 Diagnostic Codes

365.11 Primary open angle glaucoma
365.12 Low tension glaucoma
365.13 Pigmentary glaucoma
365.14 Glaucoma of childhood
365.15 Residual stage of open angle glaucoma
365.41 Glaucoma associated with chamber angle anomalies
743.20 Buphthalmos, unspecified
743.21 Simple buphthalmos
743.22 Buphthalmos associated with other ocular anomalies

Applicable HCPCS Level II Codes

A4305 Disposable drug delivery system, flow rate of 50 ml or greater per hour
A4306 Disposable drug delivery system, flow rate of 5 ml or less per hour
A4550 Surgical tray

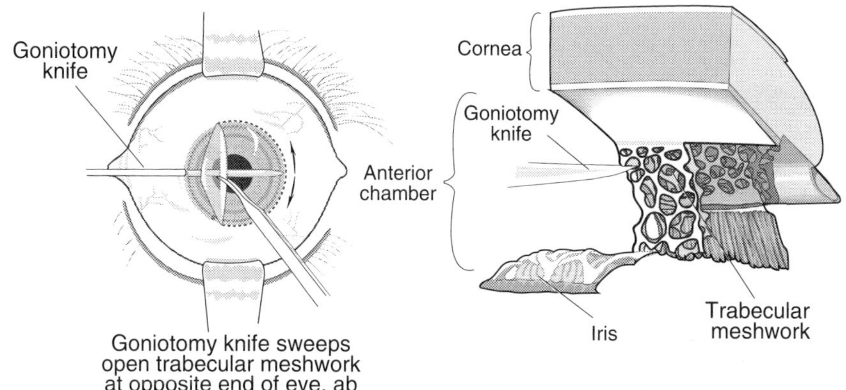

GONIOTOMY

65850 CPT CODE

CPT Description

Trabeculotomy ab externo

Explanation

Though constantly flushed and renewed, the overall pressure of aqueous is constant in a healthy eye's anterior chamber. Too little or too much fluid can cause permanent damage. To improve drainage of fluids in the eye, the physician inserts a special tool called a trabeculotome into Schlemm's canal and rotates it into the anterior chamber to open the ring of meshlike tissue (the trebecular meshwork). The name ab externo, meaning outside the eye, refers to the surgical approach from outside the eye cutting toward the anterior chamber.

Comments

If tissue is removed in this procedure, report 66170. If the trabecular meshwork is approached from across the anterior segment instead of from outside the eye, report 65820. A gonioscopy is performed for this procedure and can be reported separately with 92020. This procedure is generally performed with a subconjunctival or retrobulbar injection rather than general anesthesia.

Commonly Associated ICD•9 Procedural Codes

12.54 Trabeculotomy ab externo

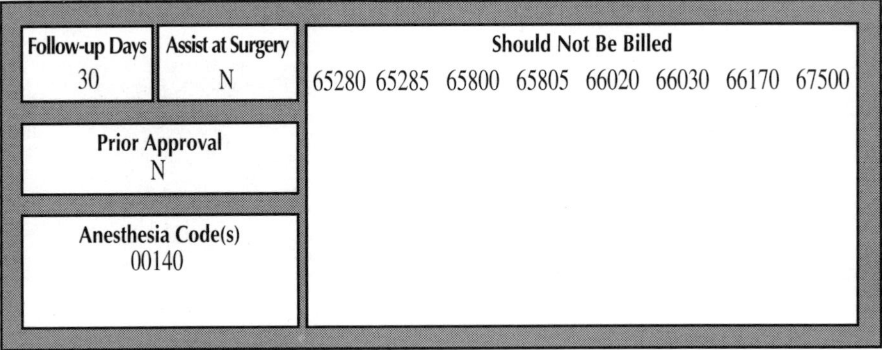

Follow-up Days	Assist at Surgery	Should Not Be Billed
30	N	65280 65285 65800 65805 66020 66030 66170 67500

Prior Approval
N

Anesthesia Code(s)
00140

Commonly Associated ICD•9 Diagnostic Codes

365.10 Open-angle glaucoma, unspecified
365.11 Primary open angle glaucoma
365.12 Low tension glaucoma
365.13 Pigmentary glaucoma
365.14 Glaucoma of childhood
365.15 Residual stage of open angle glaucoma
365.41 Glaucoma associated with chamber angle anomalies
365.60 Glaucoma associated with unspecified ocular disorder
371.11 Anterior corneal pigmentations
371.12 Stromal corneal pigmentations

Applicable HCPCS Level II Codes

A4305 Disposable drug delivery system, flow rate of 50 ml or greater per hour
A4306 Disposable drug delivery system, flow rate of 5 ml or less per hour
A4550 Surgical tray

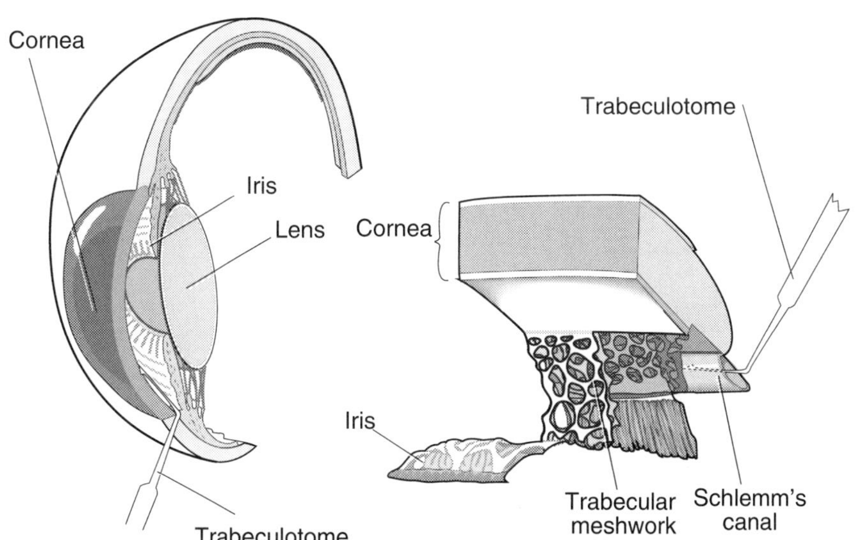

65855 CPT CODE

CPT Description

Trabeculoplasty by laser surgery, one or more sessions (defined treatment series)

Explanation

The physician uses an argon laser to selectively burn the ring of meshlike tissue at the iris-scleral junction (the trabecular meshwork) to improve the drainage of fluids in the anterior segment. The physician begins by placing a special contact on the eye to be treated. This lens allows the physician to view the angle structures of the eye and the trabecular network while using the laser. Though the trabecular network runs along the entire circumference of the iris, the physician burns holes in only a portion of that circumference during a single treatment session. In this way, the physician can measure the effects of each treatment upon the eye's fluid, and suspend treatment once the proper intraocular fluid pressure is reached. No incision is made during this procedure.

Comments

The series of treatments is reported once with the single code. If retreatment is necessary, a new treatment series should be reported with a modifier. A gonioscopy is performed for this procedure and can be reported separately with 92020. This procedure is generally performed with a topical anesthetic rather than general anesthesia.

Commonly Associated ICD•9 Procedural Codes

12.59 Other facilitation of intraocular circulation

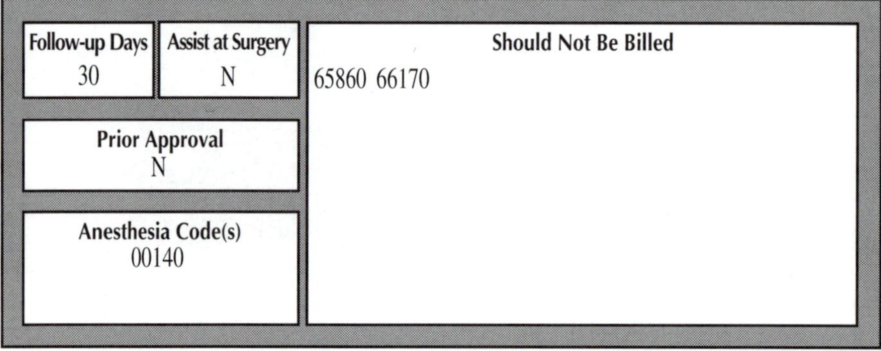

Follow-up Days	Assist at Surgery	Should Not Be Billed
30	N	65860 66170

Prior Approval
N

Anesthesia Code(s)
00140

Commonly Associated ICD•9 Diagnostic Codes

365.01 Open angle with borderline glaucoma findings
365.10 Open-angle glaucoma, unspecified
365.11 Primary open angle glaucoma
365.13 Pigmentary glaucoma
365.15 Residual stage of open angle glaucoma
365.52 Pseudoexfoliation glaucoma
365.60 Glaucoma associated with unspecified ocular disorder

Applicable HCPCS Level II Codes

A4305 Disposable drug delivery system, flow rate of 50 ml or greater per hour
A4306 Disposable drug delivery system, flow rate of 5 ml or less per hour
A4550 Surgical tray

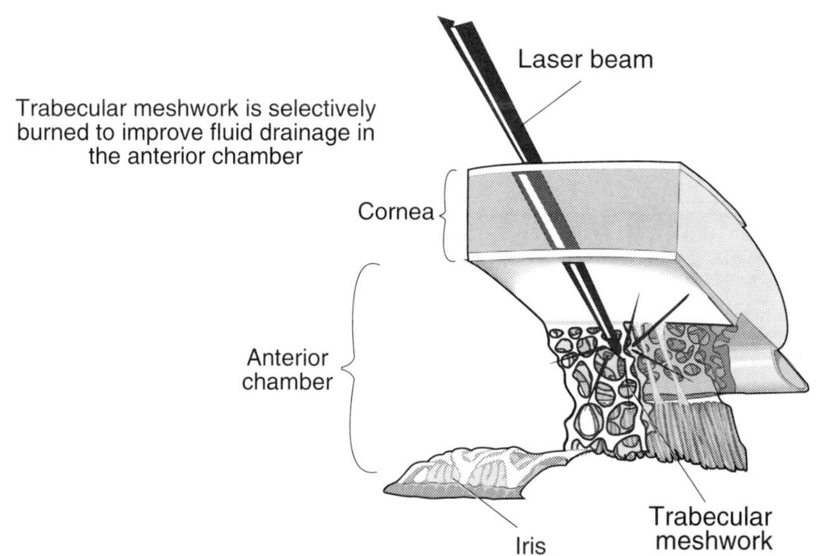

TRABECULOPLASTY

65860 CPT CODE

CPT Description

Severing adhesions of anterior segment, laser technique (separate procedure)

Explanation

Sometimes scar tissue or adhesions bind structures within the eye, interfering with vision or with intraocular pressure. The physician uses a YAG laser to selectively sever vitreal, corneal, or ciliary strands or adhesions binding the iris to adjunct structures and interfering with vision. The physician begins by placing a special contact on the eye to be treated. This lens allows the physician to view the angle structures of the eye and the trabecular network while using the laser. The strands or adhesions are not removed; they simply fall out of the visual field.

Comments

This code is a separate procedure, and by definition is usually a component of a more complex procedure. It is only reported when performed independently for a specific purpose. This procedure is generally performed with a topical anesthetic rather than general anesthesia.

Commonly Associated ICD•9 Procedural Codes

12.39 Other iridoplasty

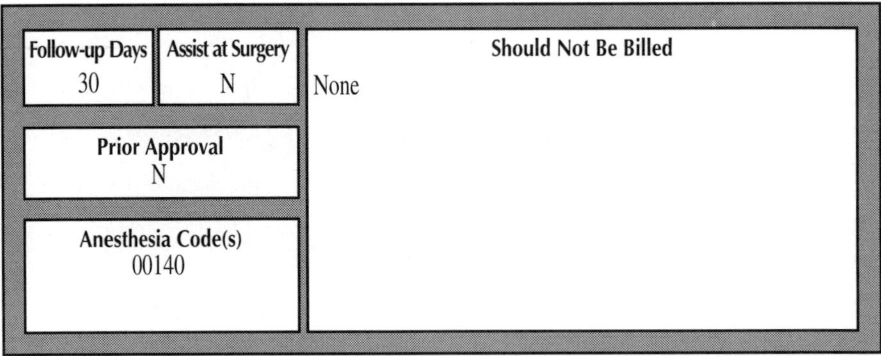

Follow-up Days	Assist at Surgery
30	N

Prior Approval
N

Anesthesia Code(s)
00140

Should Not Be Billed
None

Commonly Associated ICD•9 Diagnostic Codes

362.53 Cystoid macular degeneration of retina
364.70 Adhesions of iris, unspecified
364.72 Anterior synechiae of iris

Applicable HCPCS Level II Codes

A4305 Disposable drug delivery system, flow rate of 50 ml or greater per hour
A4306 Disposable drug delivery system, flow rate of 5 ml or less per hour
A4550 Surgical tray

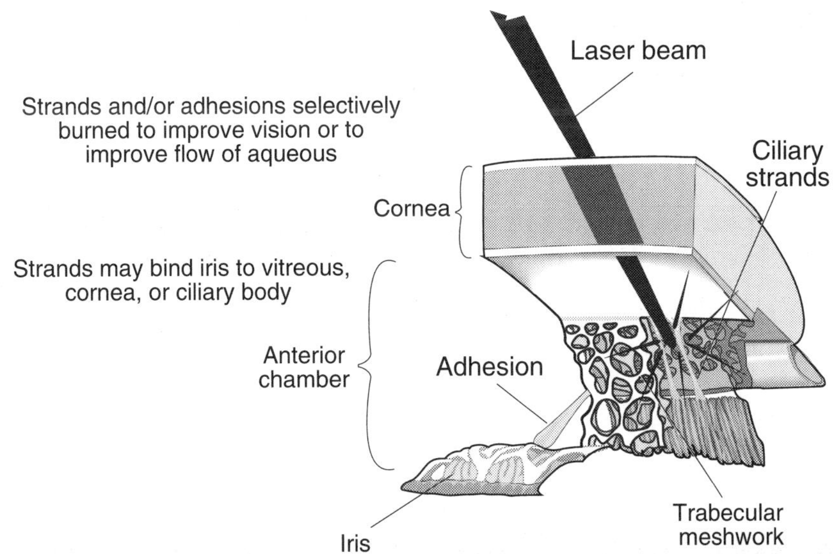

SEVERING ANTERIOR ADHESIONS

65865 CPT CODE

CPT Description

Severing adhesions of anterior segment of eye, incisional technique (with or without injection of air or liquid) (separate procedure); goniosynechiae

Explanation

Sometimes scar tissue or adhesions bind structures within the eye, interfering with vision or with intraocular pressure.Through an incision in the corneal-scleral juncture (the limbus) the physician enters the anterior segment to sever vitreal, corneal, or ciliary strands or adhesions binding the iris to adjunct structures interfering with vision. The strands or adhesions are not removed; they simply fall out of the visual field.

Comments

Code with caution: laser surgery has largely replaced this procedure. For laser surgery, see 66821. This code is a separate procedure, and by definition is usually a component of a more complex procedure. It is only reported when performed independently for a specific purpose.

Commonly Associated ICD•9 Procedural Codes

12.31 Lysis of goniosynechiae

Follow-up Days	Assist at Surgery	Should Not Be Billed
30	N	65275 65280 65800 65805 65815 65860 65930 66020 66030 66250 66500 67500

Prior Approval
N

Anesthesia Code(s)
00140

Commonly Associated ICD•9 Diagnostic Codes

364.01 Primary iridocyclitis
364.02 Recurrent iridocyclitis
364.1 Chronic iridocyclitis
364.70 Adhesions of iris, unspecified
364.71 Posterior synechiae of iris
364.72 Anterior synechiae of iris
364.73 Goniosynechiae
365.23 Chronic angle-closure glaucoma

Applicable HCPCS Level II Codes

A4305 Disposable drug delivery system, flow rate of 50 ml or greater per hour
A4306 Disposable drug delivery system, flow rate of 5 ml or less per hour
A4550 Surgical tray

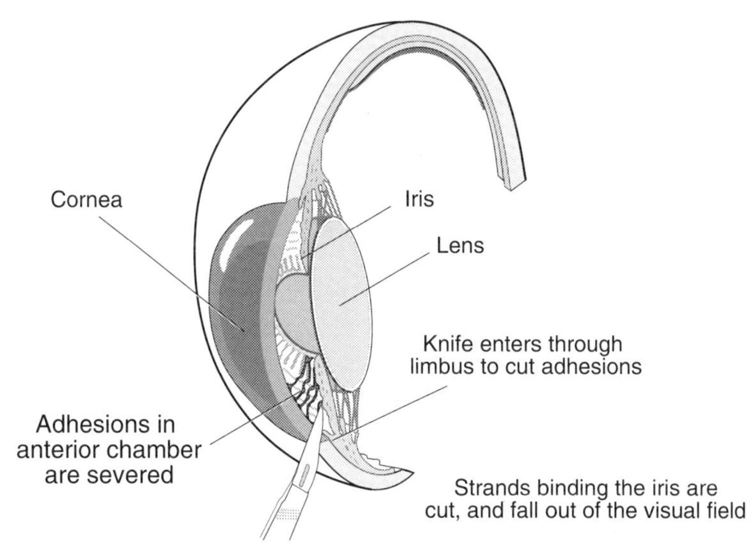

SEVERING ADHESIONS

CPT Description

65870 Severing adhesions of anterior segment of eye, incisional technique (with or without injection of air or liquid) (separate procedure); anterior synechiae, except goniosynechiae

65875 posterior synechiae

Explanation

The physician enters the anterior segment through the limbus to sever strands or adhesions binding the iris to adjunct structures interfering with vision. In the anterior synechiae (e.g., for 65870) the physician severs adhesions of the base of the iris to the cornea. For posterior synechiae (e.g., for 65875), the adhesions between the iris to the capsule of the lens or to the surface of the vitreous body are severed. Once the adhesions have been severed, the intraocular pressure may be restored with an injection of fluid or air. The incision is closed and an antibiotic and pressure patch may be applied.

Comments

Code with caution: these procedures have largely been replaced by laser surgery. For laser surgery, see 66821. These codes are separate procedures, and by definition are usually a component of a more complex procedure. Either is only reported when performed independently for a specific purpose.

Commonly Associated ICD•9 Procedural Codes

12.32 Lysis of other anterior synechiae

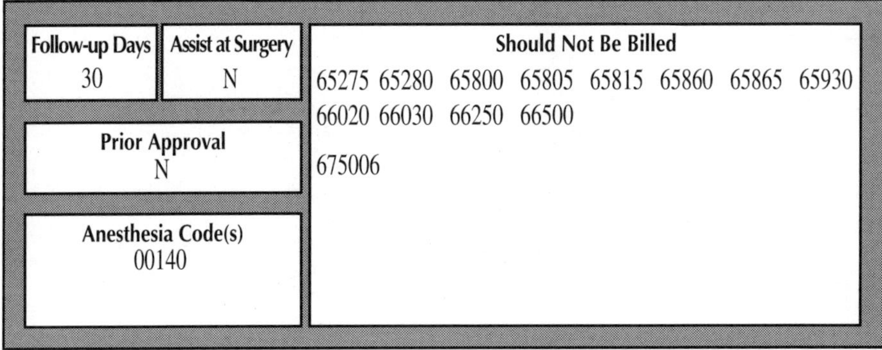

Follow-up Days	Assist at Surgery	Should Not Be Billed
30	N	65275 65280 65800 65805 65815 65860 65865 65930 66020 66030 66250 66500
Prior Approval		675006
N		
Anesthesia Code(s)		
00140		

Commonly Associated ICD•9 Diagnostic Codes

364.70 Adhesions of iris, unspecified
364.72 Anterior synechiae of iris

For 65875:

364.71 Posterior synechiae of iris
364.73 Goniosynechiae

Applicable HCPCS Level II Codes

A4305 Disposable drug delivery system, flow rate of 50 ml or greater per hour
A4306 Disposable drug delivery system, flow rate of 5 ml or less per hour
A4550 Surgical tray

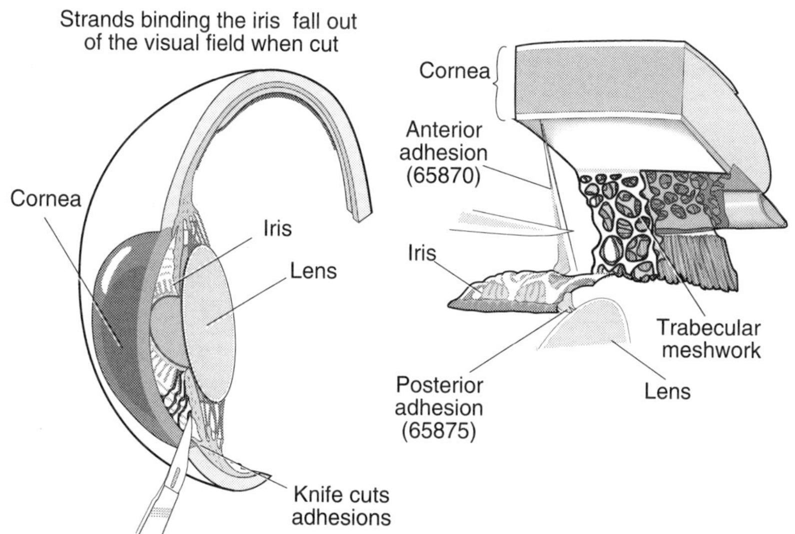

Severing Adhesions

65880 CPT CODE

CPT Description

Severing adhesions of anterior segment of eye, incisional technique (with or without injection of air or liquid) (separate procedure); corneovitreal adhesions

Explanation

The physician enters the anterior segment through the limbus to sever strands or adhesions binding the cornea to the gel-like vitreous that has prolapsed into the anterior chamber. Once the adhesions have been severed, the intraocular pressure may be restored with an injection of fluid or air. The incision is closed and an antibiotic and pressure patch may be applied.

Comments

For laser surgery, see 66821. This code is a separate procedure, and by definition is usually a component of a more complex procedure. It is only reported when performed independently for a specific purpose.

Commonly Associated ICD•9 Procedural Codes

12.34 Lysis of corneovitreal adhesions

Follow-up Days	Assist at Surgery	Should Not Be Billed
30	N	65275 65280 65800 65805 65815 65860 65870 65875 65930 66020 66030 66250 66500 67500
Prior Approval N		
Anesthesia Code(s) 00140		

Commonly Associated ICD•9 Diagnostic Codes

362.53 Cystoid macular degeneration of retina
364.70 Adhesions of iris, unspecified
364.71 Posterior synechiae of iris
364.72 Anterior synechiae of iris
364.73 Goniosynechiae
379.31 Aphakia

Applicable HCPCS Level II Codes

A4305 Disposable drug delivery system, flow rate of 50 ml or greater per hour
A4306 Disposable drug delivery system, flow rate of 5 ml or less per hour
A4550 Surgical tray

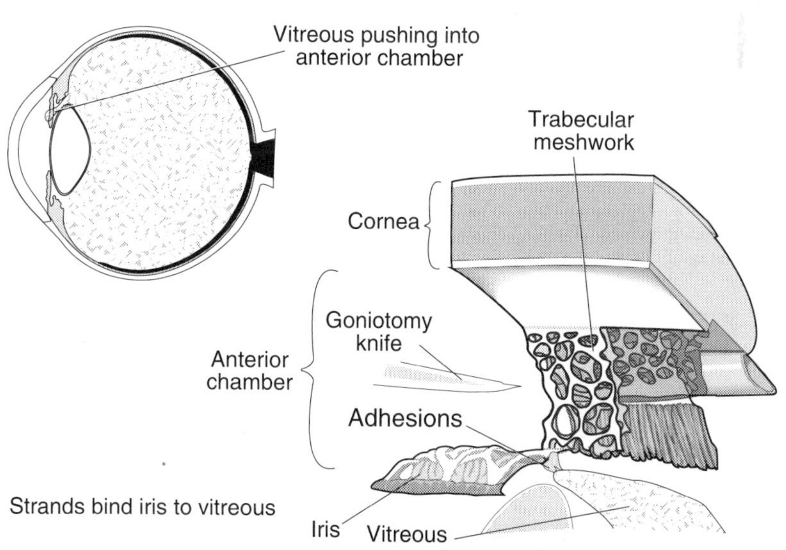

Severing Adhesions

CPT Description

Removal of epithelial downgrowth, anterior chamber eye

Explanation

Epithelial downgrowth describes the improper healing of surgical or traumatic wound to the cornea. The outer lining of the cornea (the epithelium) fails to close properly over the wound, instead growing around to the inner side of the cornea, sometimes continuing its growth to other structures of the eye. Disturbances in intraocular pressure and vision can result. The physician retracts the patient's eyelids with an ocular speculum. The physician locates and excises the extraneous epithelial tissue from where it has spread into the anterior chamber. The original wound may be trimmed and revised. Injections may be required to restore pressure in the anterior or posterior chambers. The procedure may require sutures or tissue glue, antibiotic ointment or a pressure patch.

Comments

This procedure is generally performed with a subconjunctival or retrobulbar injection rather than general anesthesia.

Commonly Associated ICD•9 Procedural Codes

12.93 Removal or destruction of epithelial downgrowth from anterior chamber

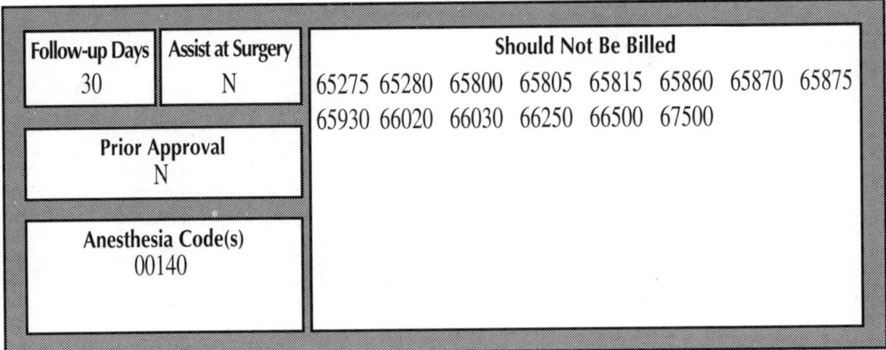

Follow-up Days	Assist at Surgery
30	N

Prior Approval
N

Anesthesia Code(s)
00140

Should Not Be Billed
65275 65280 65800 65805 65815 65860 65870 65875
65930 66020 66030 66250 66500 67500

Commonly Associated ICD•9 Diagnostic Codes

371.70 Corneal deformity, unspecified

371.89 Other corneal disorders

E878.4 Other restorative surgery causing abnormal patient reaction, or later complication, without mention of misadventure at time of operation

Applicable HCPCS Level II Codes

A4305 Disposable drug delivery system, flow rate of 50 ml or greater per hour

A4306 Disposable drug delivery system, flow rate of 5 ml or less per hour

A4550 Surgical tray

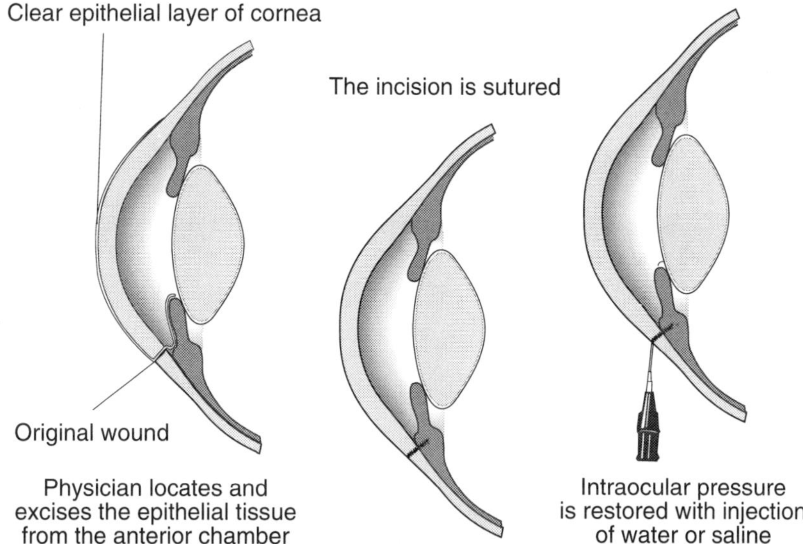

SEVERING ADHESIONS

65920 CPT CODE

CPT Description

Removal of implanted material, anterior segment eye

Explanation

The clouding of the lens capsule (cataract) causes visual loss. To correct this problem, a bad lens is replaced with an artificial one. Sometimes complications require the removal of the artificial lens. The physician retracts the patient's eyelids with an ocular speculum. The physician cuts and retracts the conjunctiva and makes an incision at the juncture of the cornea and sclera (the limbus). The physician removes from the anterior segment the previously placed artificial lens (called an intraocular lens or IOL). It is not replaced. The limbus and the conjunctiva are closed with sutures. Antibiotic or a pressure patch may be applied.

Comments

This code is also used if the physician amputates the haptic of an anterior chamber lens. If the old lens is replaced with a new one, use 66986.

Commonly Associated ICD•9 Procedural Codes

13.8 Removal of implanted lens

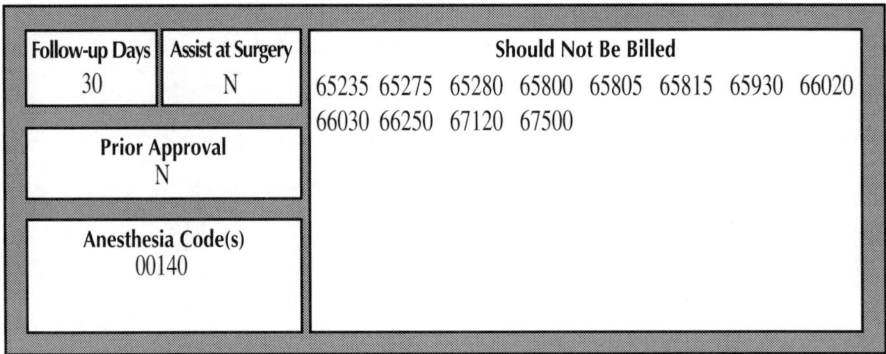

Follow-up Days	Assist at Surgery	Should Not Be Billed
30	N	65235 65275 65280 65800 65805 65815 65930 66020 66030 66250 67120 67500

Prior Approval
N

Anesthesia Code(s)
00140

Commonly Associated ICD•9 Diagnostic Codes

364.04 Secondary iridocyclitis, noninfectious
364.41 Hyphema of iris and ciliary body
365.9 Unspecified glaucoma
996.53 Mechanical complication of ocular lens prosthesis
996.69 Infection and inflammatory reaction due to other internal prosthetic device, implant, and graft
V43.1 Lens replaced by other means

Applicable HCPCS Level II Codes

A4305 Disposable drug delivery system, flow rate of 50 ml or greater per hour
A4306 Disposable drug delivery system, flow rate of 5 ml or less per hour
A4550 Surgical tray

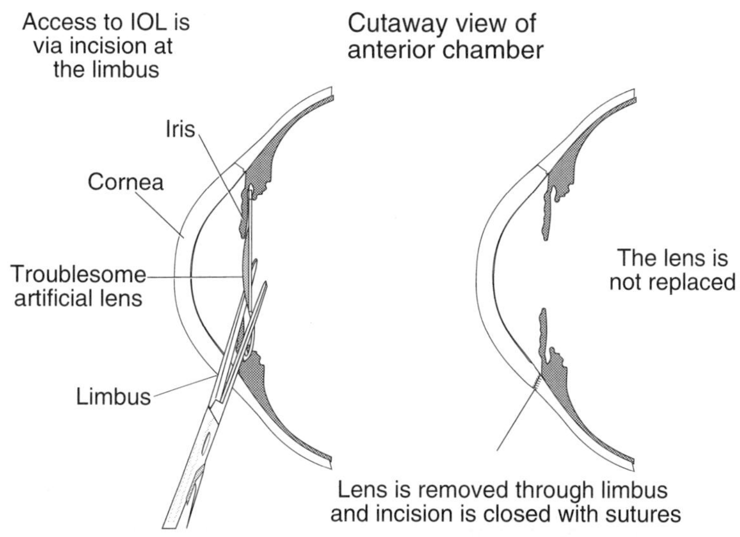

65930 CPT CODE

CPT Description

Removal of blood clot, anterior segment eye

Explanation

A blood clot in the anterior segment can block the flow of aqueous, thereby elevating intraocular pressure. It can also stain the cornea. Either condition can lead to permanent visual loss. The physician retracts the patient's eyelids with an ocular speculum. The physician uses a needle to aspirate a blood clot which has pooled in the anterior section between the iris and the cornea. The needle may enter the anterior segment through the cornea or through the limbus (the juncture of the cornea and sclera). Topical antibiotic or a patch may be applied when the procedure is complete.

Comments

If blood, but not a clot, is removed from the eye, use 65815. This procedure is generally performed with a subconjunctival or retrobulbar injection rather than general anesthesia.

Commonly Associated ICD•9 Procedural Codes

12.91 Therapeutic evacuation of anterior chamber

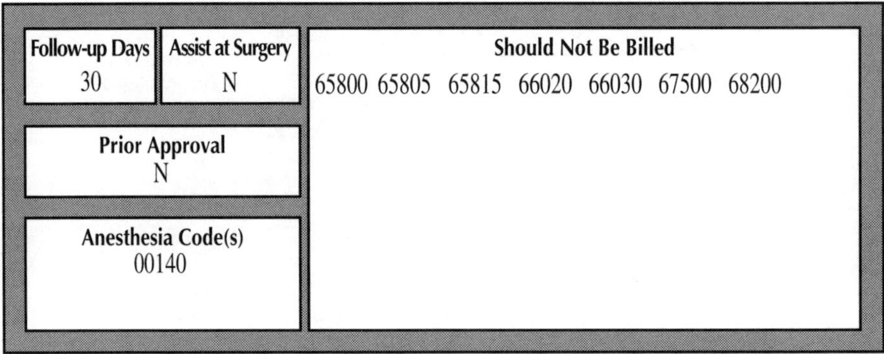

Follow-up Days	Assist at Surgery
30	N

Prior Approval
N

Anesthesia Code(s)
00140

Should Not Be Billed
65800 65805 65815 66020 66030 67500 68200

Commonly Associated ICD•9 Diagnostic Codes

364.41 Hyphema of iris and ciliary body
365.65 Glaucoma associated with ocular trauma
921.3 Contusion of eyeball

Applicable HCPCS Level II Codes

A4305 Disposable drug delivery system, flow rate of 50 ml or greater per hour
A4306 Disposable drug delivery system, flow rate of 5 ml or less per hour
A4550 Surgical tray

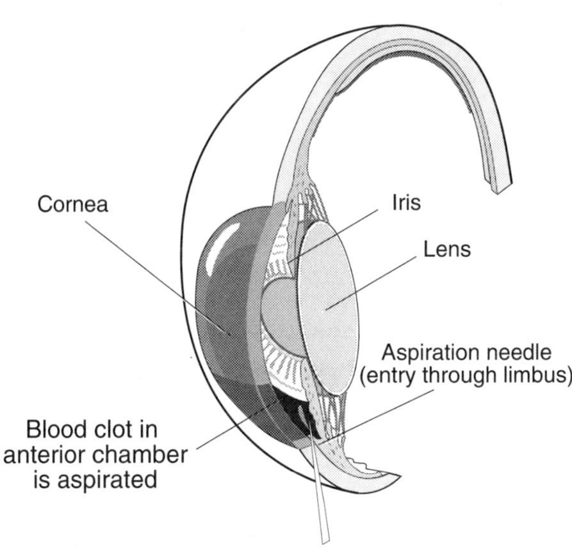

Blood Clot Removal

CPT Description

66020 Injection, anterior chamber (separate procedure); air or liquid

66030 medication

Explanation

Though constantly flushed and renewed, the overall pressure of aqueous is constant in a healthy eye's anterior chamber. Too little or too much fluid can cause permanent damage. The physician administers a needle injection of air or liquid (e.g., 66020) or medication (e.g., 66030) to the anterior of the eye. The needle may enter the anterior segment through the cornea or through the limbus (the juncture of the cornea and sclera).

Comments

These codes are separate procedures, and by definition are usually a component of more complex procedures. They are only reported when performed independently for a specific purpose. Also, 66030 is a starred procedure reporting the surgical service only. Any pre- or postoperative services should be reported also. These procedures are generally performed with topical anesthetic rather than general anesthesia.

Commonly Associated ICD•9 Procedural Codes

12.92 Injection into anterior chamber

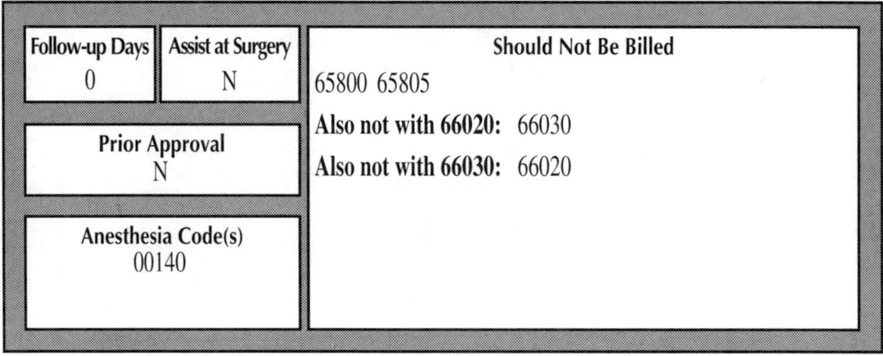

Follow-up Days	Assist at Surgery
0	N

Prior Approval
N

Anesthesia Code(s)
00140

Should Not Be Billed

65800 65805

Also not with 66020: 66030

Also not with 66030: 66020

Commonly Associated ICD•9 Diagnostic Codes

364.73 Goniosynechiae
365.22 Acute angle-closure glaucoma

Applicable HCPCS Level II Codes

A4305 Disposable drug delivery system, flow rate of 50 ml or greater per hour
A4306 Disposable drug delivery system, flow rate of 5 ml or less per hour
A4550 Surgical tray

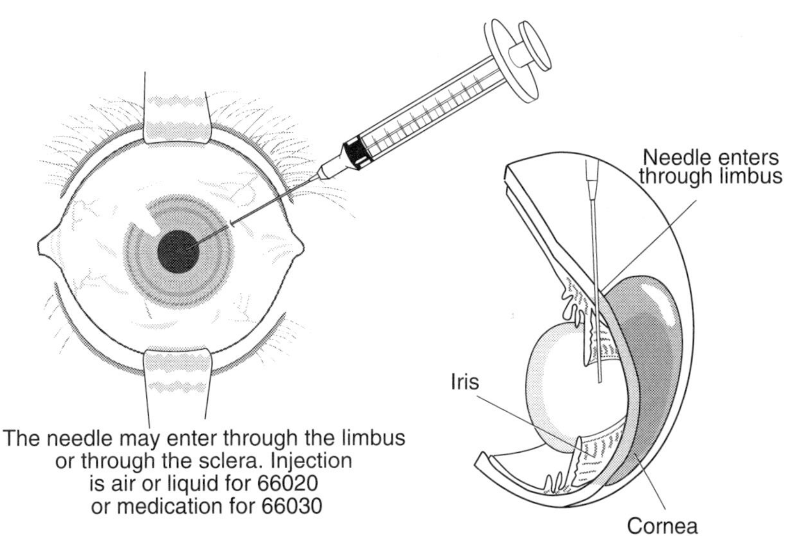

The needle may enter through the limbus or through the sclera. Injection is air or liquid for 66020 or medication for 66030

ANTERIOR SEGMENT INJECTION

66130 CPT CODE

CPT Description

Excision of lesion, sclera

Explanation

The sclera, coming from the Greek word for "hard," is the tough, white, outer coat of the eye. To remove a scleral lesion, the physician cuts through the thin, transparent conjunctiva and then snips the lesion with scleral scissors. The scleral and conjunctival wounds may not require sutures. The physician then applies antibiotic ointment and possibly a 24-hour pressure patch.

Comments

Report 99000 if the specimen is taken to an outside laboratory for biopsy. This procedure is generally performed with a subconjunctival injection or topical anesthetic rather than general anesthesia. For operations on posterior sclera, see 67250 and 67255.

Commonly Associated ICD•9 Procedural Codes

12.84 Excision or destruction of lesion of sclera

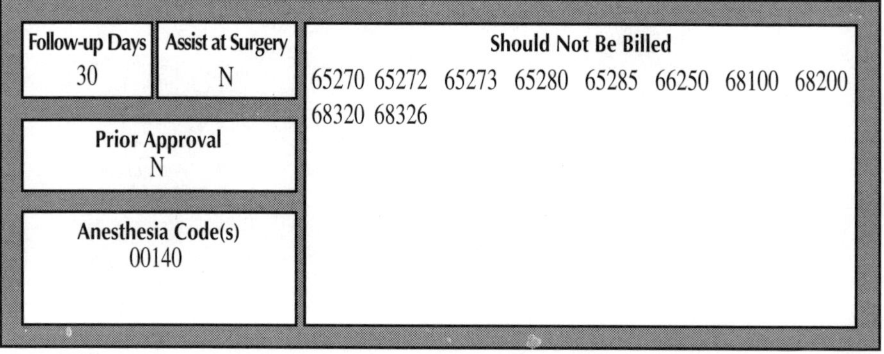

Follow-up Days	Assist at Surgery
30	N

Prior Approval
N

Anesthesia Code(s)
00140

Should Not Be Billed
65270 65272 65273 65280 65285 66250 68100 68200 68320 68326

Commonly Associated ICD•9 Diagnostic Codes

190.0 Malignant neoplasm of eyeball, except conjunctiva, cornea, retina, and choroid
224.0 Benign neoplasm of eyeball, except conjunctiva, cornea, retina, and choroid

Applicable HCPCS Level II Codes

A4305 Disposable drug delivery system, flow rate of 50 ml or greater per hour
A4306 Disposable drug delivery system, flow rate of 5 ml or less per hour
A4550 Surgical tray

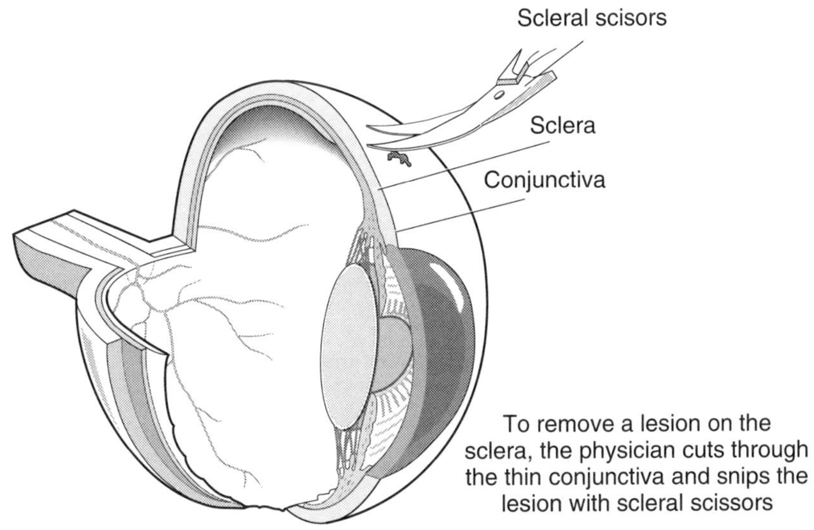

LESION EXCISION

CPT Description

66150 Fistulization of sclera for glaucoma; trephination with iridectomy

66155 thermocauterization with iridectomy

Explanation

Though constantly flushed and renewed, the overall pressure of aqueous is constant in a healthy eye's anterior chamber. Too little or too much fluid can cause permanent damage. To create a new pathway for fluids in the eye, the physician makes an incision in the conjunctiva near the limbus (the corneal-scleral juncture). Either by using a trephine to remove a circular portion of sclera and iris (e.g., 65150), or by destroying a portion of the sclera and iris by burning it with a hot probe (e.g., 65155), the physician creates a collection area to improve the flow of aqueous. One method of this procedure is called Elliot's operation. The physician closes the incision with sutures and may restore the intraocular pressure with an injection of water or saline. A topical antibiotic or pressure patch may be applied.

Comments

Use 66150 with caution; this procedure is rarely performed. For operations on posterior sclera, see 67250 and 67235. This procedure is generally performed with a subconjunctival injection or topical anesthetic rather than general anesthesia.

Commonly Associated ICD•9 Procedural Codes

12.61 Trephination of sclera with iridectomy

12.62 Thermocauterization of sclera with iridectomy

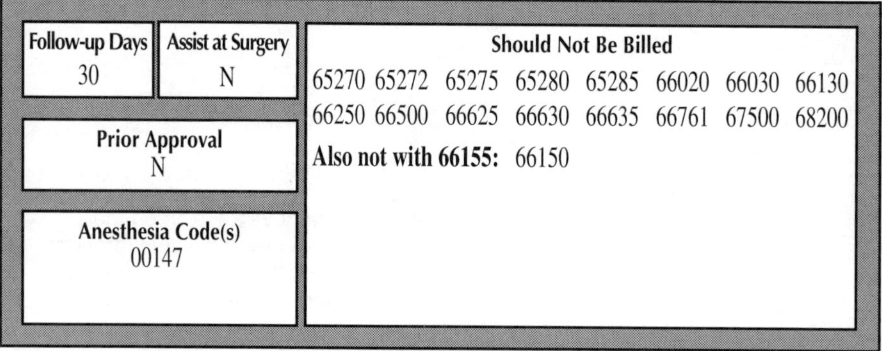

Follow-up Days	Assist at Surgery
30	N

Prior Approval
N

Anesthesia Code(s)
00147

Should Not Be Billed

65270 65272 65275 65280 65285 66020 66030 66130
66250 66500 66625 66630 66635 66761 67500 68200

Also not with 66155: 66150

Commonly Associated ICD•9 Diagnostic Codes

365.20 Primary angle-closure glaucoma, unspecified
365.21 Intermittent angle-closure glaucoma
365.22 Acute angle-closure glaucoma
365.23 Chronic angle-closure glaucoma
365.24 Residual stage of angle-closure glaucoma
365.42 Glaucoma associated with anomalies of iris
365.51 Phacolytic glaucoma
365.52 Pseudoexfoliation glaucoma

Applicable HCPCS Level II Codes

A4305 Disposable drug delivery system, flow rate of 50 ml or greater per hour
A4306 Disposable drug delivery system, flow rate of 5 ml or less per hour
A4550 Surgical tray

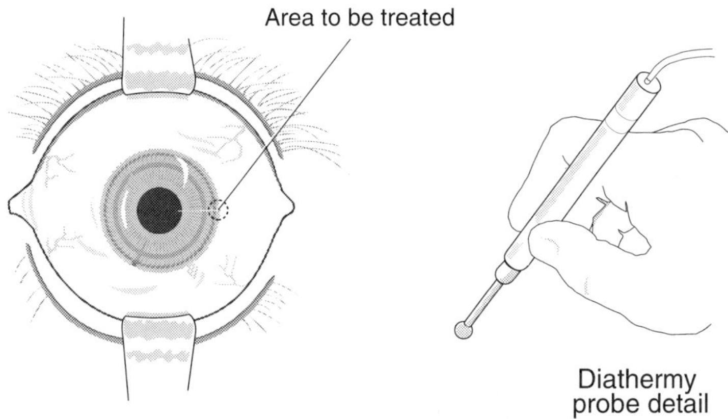

If a trephine is used to create the fistula, report 66150
If thermocauterization is applied, report 66155

CPT Description

Fistulization of sclera for glaucoma; sclerectomy with punch or scissors, with iridectomy

Explanation

Though constantly flushed and renewed, the overall pressure of aqueous is constant in a healthy eye's anterior chamber. Too little or too much fluid can cause permanent damage. To improve the flow of aqueous, the physician makes an incision in the conjunctiva near the limbus (the corneal-scleral juncture). By using a punch or scleral scissors, the physician removes a portion of sclera and iris, creating a collection area for fluids in the anterior chamber. Various methods of sclerectomy include Lindner's, LaGrange, Knapp's, Holth's and Herbert's operations. The physician closes the incision with sutures and may restore the intraocular pressure with an injection of water or saline. A topical antibiotic or pressure patch may be applied.

Comments

For operations on posterior sclera, see 67250 and 67235. This procedure is generally performed with a subconjunctival or retrobulbar injection rather than general anesthesia.

Commonly Associated ICD•9 Procedural Codes

12.65 Other scleral fistulization with iridectomy

Follow-up Days	Assist at Surgery
30	N

Prior Approval
N

Anesthesia Code(s)
00147

Should Not Be Billed

65270 65272 65273 65275 65280 65285 65815 65930
66020 66030 66130 66150 66250 66500 66600 66625
66630 66635 67500 68200 68320 68326

Commonly Associated ICD•9 Diagnostic Codes

365.20 Primary angle-closure glaucoma, unspecified
365.21 Intermittent angle-closure glaucoma
365.22 Acute angle-closure glaucoma
365.23 Chronic angle-closure glaucoma
365.24 Residual stage of angle-closure glaucoma
365.42 Glaucoma associated with anomalies of iris
365.51 Phacolytic glaucoma
365.52 Pseudoexfoliation glaucoma

Applicable HCPCS Level II Codes

A4305 Disposable drug delivery system, flow rate of 50 ml or greater per hour
A4306 Disposable drug delivery system, flow rate of 5 ml or less per hour
A4550 Surgical tray

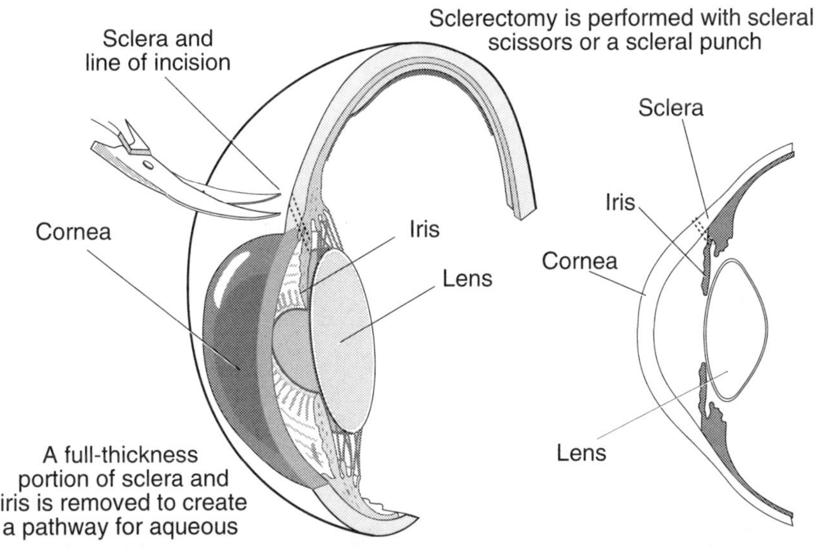

Sclerectomy

CPT Description

Fistulization of sclera for glaucoma; iridencleisis or iridotasis

Explanation

Though constantly flushed and renewed, the overall pressure of aqueous is constant in a healthy eye's anterior chamber. Too little or too much fluid can cause permanent damage. To improve the flow of fluids in the eye, the physician places an ocular speculum in the patient's eye, and accesses the anterior chamber through an incision through the limbus (the corneal-scleral juncture). The physician creates a permanent drainage route through the anterior chamber by taking a piece of iris tissue clipped with scleral scissors from the edge of the iris and wedging it into an incision in the iris so that it will act as a wick to draw aqueous from one side of the iris to the other. The physician closes the incision with sutures and may restore the intraocular pressure with an injection of water or saline. A topical antibiotic or pressure patch may be applied.

Comments

Code with caution: this procedure is more of historic value than practical significance. It has largely been abandoned. Include a cover letter. This procedure would generally be performed with a subconjunctival or retrobulbar injection rather than general anesthesia.

Commonly Associated ICD•9 Procedural Codes

12.63 Iridencleisis and iridotasis

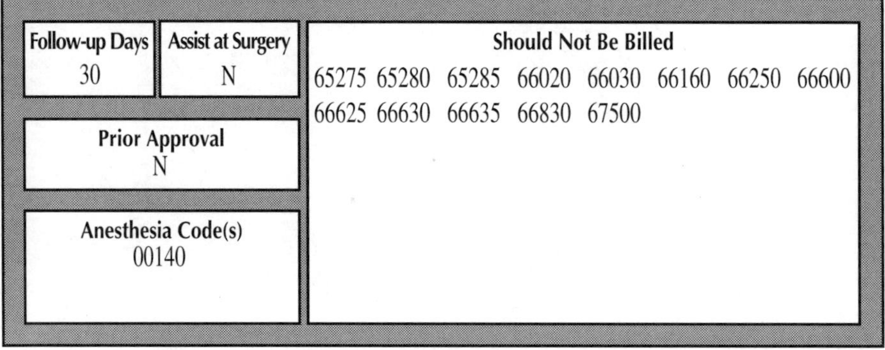

Follow-up Days	Assist at Surgery	Should Not Be Billed
30	N	65275 65280 65285 66020 66030 66160 66250 66600 66625 66630 66635 66830 67500

Prior Approval
N

Anesthesia Code(s)
00140

Commonly Associated ICD•9 Diagnostic Codes

365.20 Primary angle-closure glaucoma, unspecified
365.21 Intermittent angle-closure glaucoma
365.22 Acute angle-closure glaucoma
365.23 Chronic angle-closure glaucoma
365.24 Residual stage of angle-closure glaucoma
365.42 Glaucoma associated with anomalies of iris
365.51 Phacolytic glaucoma
365.52 Pseudoexfoliation glaucoma

Applicable HCPCS Level II Codes

A4305 Disposable drug delivery system, flow rate of 50 ml or greater per hour
A4306 Disposable drug delivery system, flow rate of 5 ml or less per hour
A4550 Surgical tray

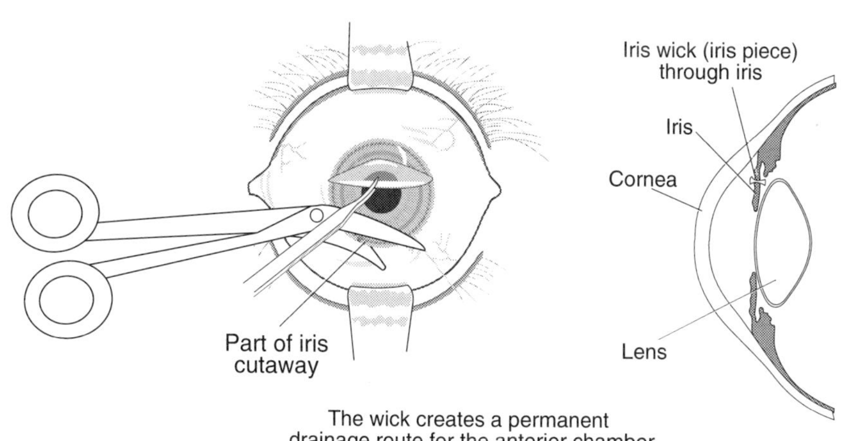

The wick creates a permanent drainage route for the anterior chamber

CPT Description

66170 Fistulization of sclera for glaucoma; trabeculectomy ab externo in absence of previous surgery

66172 trabeculectomy ab externo with scarring from previous ocular surgery or trauma (includes injection of antifibrotic agents)

Explanation

Though constantly flushed and renewed, the overall pressure of aqueous is constant in a healthy eye's anterior chamber. Too little or too much fluid can cause permanent damage. The physician places an ocular speculum in the patient's eye, and accesses the anterior chamber through an incision through the limbus (the corneal-scleral juncture).To promote better drainage of fluid, the physician removes a partial thickness portion of the ring of meshlike tissue at the iris-scleral junction (the trebecular meshwork), and a scleral trap door is left open so that aqueous may flow through the new channel into the space between the conjunctival and the sclera or cornea (bleb). The physician closes the incision with sutures and may restore the intraocular pressure with an injection of water or saline. A topical antibiotic or pressure patch may be applied. This procedure is performed in absence of previous surgery (e.g., for 66170) or as a repeated surgery where adhesions are reduced (e.g., for 66172). The adhesions may also have been caused by trauma.

Comments

These codes are new or revised in 1994. This procedure is nearly identical to 65850 with two exceptions: The scleral dissection is shallower here and the full thickness wedge of trabecular meshwork is removed here rather than simply opened. This procedure is generally performed with a subconjunctival or retrobulbar injection rather than general anesthesia. Any antimetabolite injection associated with this procedure may be separately reported.

Commonly Associated ICD•9 Procedural Codes

12.64 Trabeculectomy ab externo

Follow-up Days	Assist at Surgery	Should Not Be Billed
30	N	65275 65280 65286 65850 66020 66030 66250 66630 66635 66635 67500

Prior Approval
N

Anesthesia Code(s)
00140

Commonly Associated ICD•9 Diagnostic Codes

365.10 Open-angle glaucoma, unspecified
365.12 Low tension glaucoma
365.13 Pigmentary glaucoma
365.14 Glaucoma of childhood
365.15 Residual stage of open angle glaucoma
365.23 Chronic angle-closure glaucoma
365.24 Residual stage of angle-closure glaucoma
365.42 Glaucoma associated with anomalies of iris
365.52 Pseudoexfoliation glaucoma

Applicable HCPCS Level II Codes

A4305 Disposable drug delivery system, flow rate of 50 ml or greater per hour
A4306 Disposable drug delivery system, flow rate of 5 ml or less per hour
A4550 Surgical tray

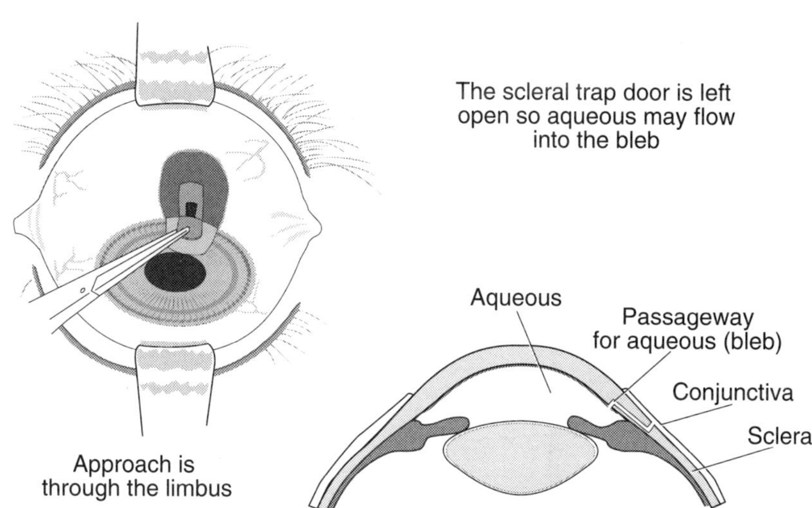

CPT Description

66180 Aqueous shunt to extraocular reservoir, (eg, Molteno, Schocket, Denver-Krupin)

66185 Revision of aqueous shunt to extraocular reservoir

Explanation

Though constantly flushed and renewed, the overall pressure of aqueous is constant in a healthy eye's anterior chamber. Too little or too much fluid can cause permanent damage. To enhance drainage, the physician places an ocular speculum in the patient's eye and makes an incision in the conjunctiva and sutures tubing to the sclera. The tubing enters the anterior portion of the eye at the juncture of the sclera and cornea (the limbus). This improves the aqueous flow in the anterior chamber. The tube implant connects to a reservoir plate (a bleb) sutured into place behind the pars plana between the extraocular muscles. The physician stretches conjunctival tissue over the shunt and reservoir and sutures it into place. The physician closes the incision with sutures and may restore the intraocular pressure with an injection of water or saline. A topical antibiotic or pressure patch may be applied. A revision is done and 66185 reported if the first procedure is unsuccessful and must be altered.

Comments

66180 is sometimes done as a two-phase procedure. If this is the case, report 66180 once. The second phase would not be considered a revision, but would be part of the original procedure. Use 66185 if the first procedure proves unsuccessful over time and must be revised. This procedure is generally performed with a subconjunctival injection rather than general anesthesia.

Commonly Associated ICD•9 Procedural Codes

12.66 Postoperative revision of scleral fistulization procedure

12.69 Other scleral fistulizing procedure

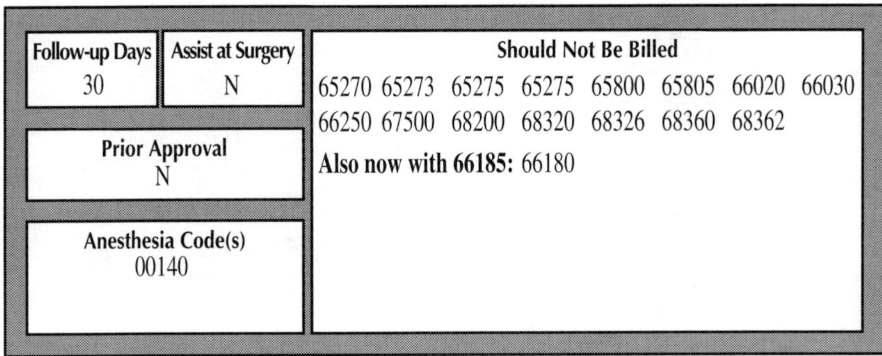

Follow-up Days	Assist at Surgery
30	N

Prior Approval
N

Anesthesia Code(s)
00140

Should Not Be Billed

65270 65273 65275 65275 65800 65805 66020 66030 66250 67500 68200 68320 68326 68360 68362

Also now with 66185: 66180

Commonly Associated ICD•9 Diagnostic Codes

365.11 Primary open angle glaucoma
365.20 Primary angle-closure glaucoma, unspecified
365.21 Intermittent angle-closure glaucoma
365.23 Chronic angle-closure glaucoma
365.24 Residual stage of angle-closure glaucoma
365.42 Glaucoma associated with anomalies of iris
365.63 Glaucoma associated with vascular disorders

Applicable HCPCS Level II Codes

A4305 Disposable drug delivery system, flow rate of 50 ml or greater per hour
A4306 Disposable drug delivery system, flow rate of 5 ml or less per hour
A4550 Surgical tray

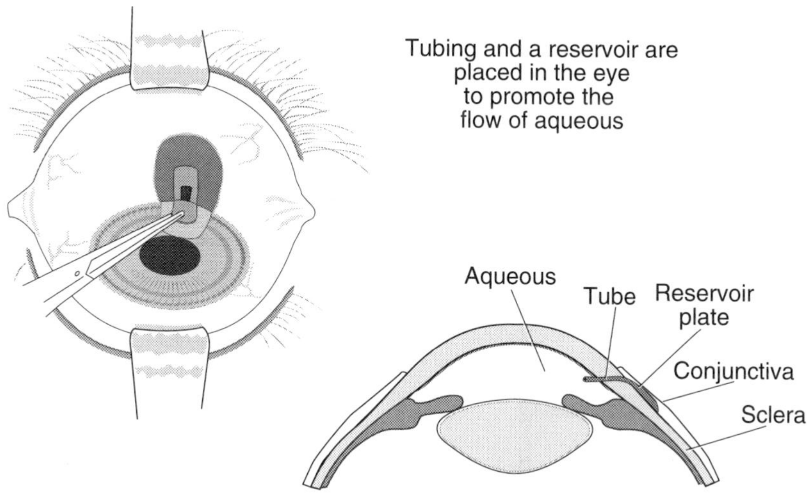

Report 66180 for the original surgery and 66185 for a revision

CPT Description

66220 Repair of scleral staphyloma; without graft

66225 with graft

Explanation

A staphyloma is a bulging protrusion of the vascular coating of the eyeball (uvea) into a thin, stretched portion of the sclera. To repair the staphyloma, the physician places an ocular speculum in the patient's eye, and makes an incision in the conjunctiva and sclera over the site of a staphyloma. The physician excises the full-thickness staphyloma. A piece of stretched sclera may also be removed. The physician uses sutures or tissue glue in the layered repair. Antibiotic ointment and a patch may be applied. A graft (e.g., 66225) usually indicates that size of the staphyloma required that donor sclera tissue be grafted across the wound.

Comments

For scleral procedures in retinal surgery, see 67120. This procedure is generally performed with a subconjunctival injection rather than general anesthesia.

Commonly Associated ICD•9 Procedural Codes

12.85 Repair of scleral staphyloma with graft

12.86 Other repair of scleral staphyloma

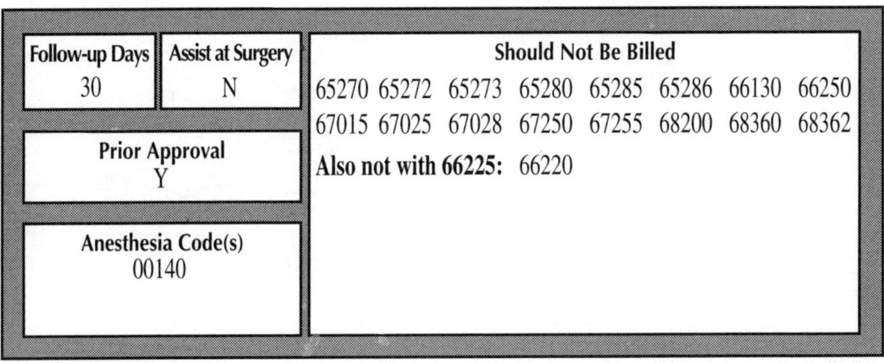

Follow-up Days	Assist at Surgery
30	N

Prior Approval
Y

Anesthesia Code(s)
00140

Should Not Be Billed

65270 65272 65273 65280 65285 65286 66130 66250
67015 67025 67028 67250 67255 68200 68360 68362

Also not with 66225: 66220

Commonly Associated ICD•9 Diagnostic Codes

379.11 Scleral ectasia
379.12 Staphyloma posticum
379.13 Equatorial staphyloma
379.14 Anterior staphyloma, localized
379.15 Ring staphyloma

Applicable HCPCS Level II Codes

A4305 Disposable drug delivery system, flow rate of 50 ml or greater per hour
A4306 Disposable drug delivery system, flow rate of 5 ml or less per hour
A4550 Surgical tray

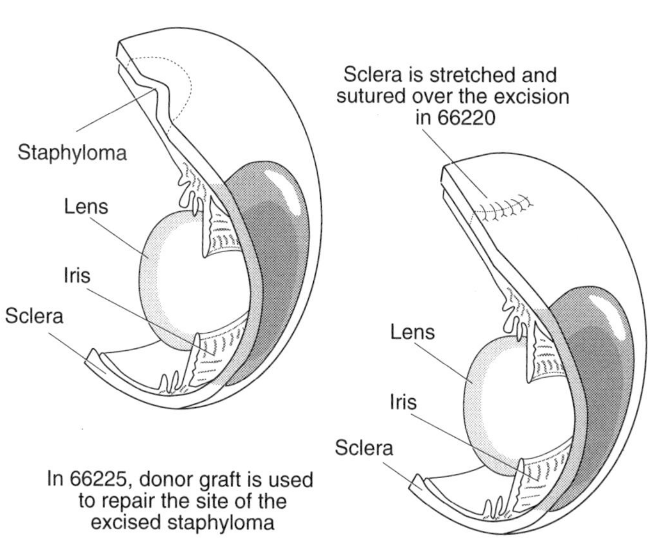

66500–66505 CPT CODES

CPT Description

66500 Iridotomy by stab incision (separate procedure); except transfixion

66505 with transfixion as for iris bombe

Explanation

Though constantly flushed and renewed, the overall pressure of aqueous is constant in a healthy eye's anterior chamber. Too little or too much fluid can cause permanent damage. To enhance the flow of fluids in the anterior chamber, the physician makes an incision in the corneal-scleral juncture (the limbus). The physician slices through the iris in a side-to-side motion in an effort to increase the flow of aqueous hampered by a pupilary block (e.g., 66500). No tissue is removed. In the iris bombe, where the iris balloons forward blocking aqueous outflow channels, the surgeon pierces the iris in two places (e.g., 66505). The physician closes the incision with sutures and may restore intraocular pressure with an injection of water or saline. A topical antibiotic or pressure patch may be applied.

Comments

No tissue is removed in this procedure. If tissue is removed, report 66600 or 66605. Note that 66500 and 66505 are separate procedures, and by definition report a service that is usually a part of a more complex procedure. However, if performed alone and for a specific purpose, they should be reported. These procedures are generally performed with a subconjunctival or retrobulbar injection rather than general anesthesia.

Commonly Associated ICD•9 Procedural Codes

12.11 Iridotomy with transfixion

12.12 Other iridotomy

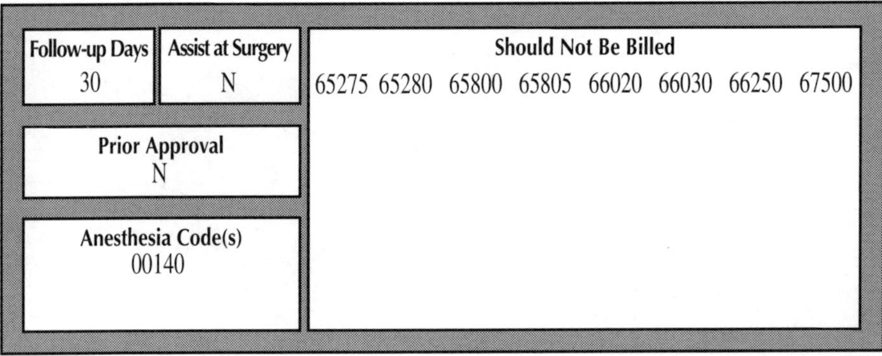

Follow-up Days	Assist at Surgery	Should Not Be Billed
30	N	65275 65280 65800 65805 66020 66030 66250 67500

Prior Approval
N

Anesthesia Code(s)
00140

Commonly Associated ICD•9 Diagnostic Codes

364.74 Adhesions and disruptions of pupillary membranes
365.20 Primary angle-closure glaucoma, unspecified
365.21 Intermittent angle-closure glaucoma
365.22 Acute angle-closure glaucoma
365.23 Chronic angle-closure glaucoma
365.24 Residual stage of angle-closure glaucoma
365.42 Glaucoma associated with anomalies of iris
365.61 Glaucoma associated with pupillary block

Applicable HCPCS Level II Codes

A4305 Disposable drug delivery system, flow rate of 50 ml or greater per hour
A4306 Disposable drug delivery system, flow rate of 5 ml or less per hour
A4550 Surgical tray

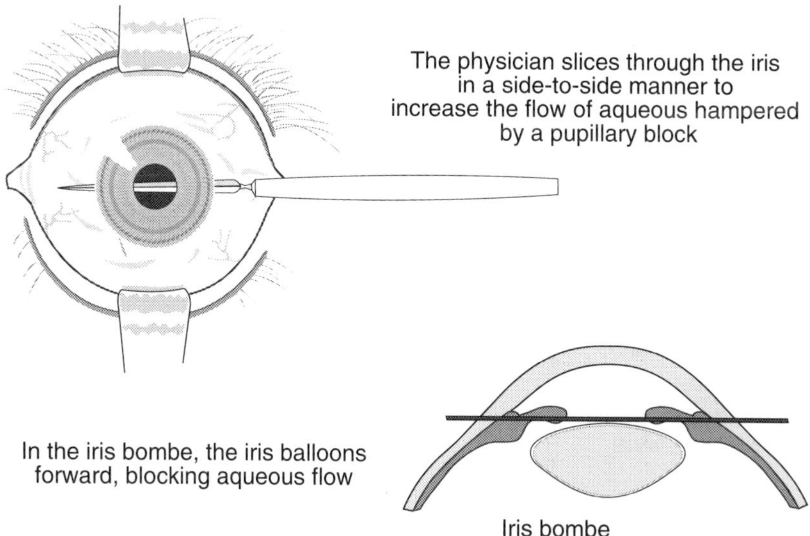

CPT Description

66600 Iridectomy, with corneoscleral or corneal section; for removal of lesion

66605 with cyclectomy

Explanation

The physician places a contact lens on the patient's eye to help direct the laser's beam. The excision of a full-thickness piece of the iris is usually accomplished with an argon laser. The physician uses the "chipping away technique" until the iris is penetrated for the excision. With cyclectomy (e.g., 66605), the burn is deeper, going through the iris into the ciliary body.

Comments

If no tissue is removed, use 66500. Report 99000 if the lesion specimen is taken to an outside laboratory for biopsy. This procedure is generally performed with a subconjunctival or retrobulbar injection rather than general anesthesia.

Commonly Associated ICD•9 Procedural Codes

12.40 Removal of lesion of anterior segment of eye, not otherwise specified

12.41 Destruction of lesion of iris, nonexcisional

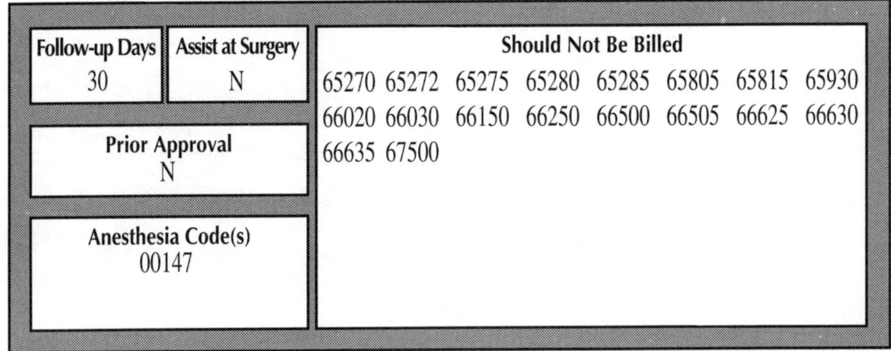

Follow-up Days	Assist at Surgery
30	N

Prior Approval
N

Anesthesia Code(s)
00147

Should Not Be Billed

65270 65272 65275 65280 65285 65805 65815 65930 66020 66030 66150 66250 66500 66505 66625 66630 66635 67500

Commonly Associated ICD•9 Diagnostic Codes

190.0 Malignant neoplasm of eyeball, except conjunctiva, cornea, retina, and choroid
224.0 Benign neoplasm of eyeball, except conjunctiva, cornea, retina, and choroid
238.8 Neoplasm of uncertain behavior of other specified sites
364.60 Idiopathic cysts of iris and ciliary body
364.62 Exudative cysts of iris or anterior chamber

Applicable HCPCS Level II Codes

A4305 Disposable drug delivery system, flow rate of 50 ml or greater per hour
A4306 Disposable drug delivery system, flow rate of 5 ml or less per hour
A4550 Surgical tray

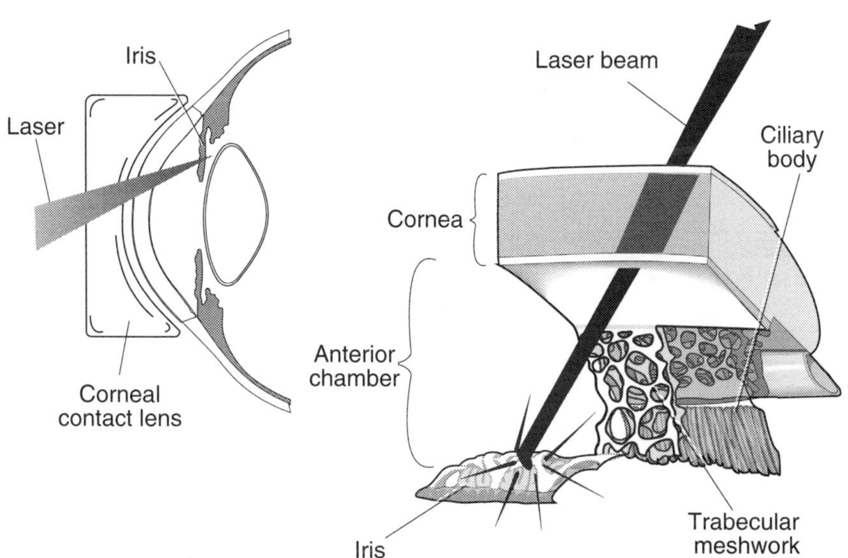

IRIDECTOMY

66625 CPT CODE

CPT Description

Iridectomy, with corneoscleral or corneal section; peripheral for glaucoma (separate procedure)

Explanation

After placing an ocular speculum in the patient's eye, the physician makes an incision at the juncture of the cornea and sclera (the limbus). The physician then removes a piece of iris, providing a direct passageway for aqueous. This causes the intraocular pressure to fall as aqueous from behind the iris can then flow forward and drain from the eye. This procedure is also called basal, buttonhole or stenopeic iridectomy. The physician may close the incision with sutures and may restore the intraocular pressure with an injection of water or saline. A topical antibiotic or pressure patch may be applied.

Comments

As a separate procedure, this procedure is usually an intrinsic part of a more complex service, and therefore is not reportable. However, when performed separately and for a specific purpose, it can be reported separately. For iridotomy, by photocoagulation, see 66761. This procedure is generally performed with a subconjunctival or retrobulbar injection rather than general anesthesia.

Commonly Associated ICD•9 Procedural Codes

12.14 Other iridectomy

Follow-up Days	Assist at Surgery
30	N

Prior Approval
N

Anesthesia Code(s)
00147

Should Not Be Billed
65275 65280 65285 65800 65805 65815 65930 66020
66030 66250 66500 66505

Commonly Associated ICD•9 Diagnostic Codes

364.74 Adhesions and disruptions of pupillary membranes
365.20 Primary angle-closure glaucoma, unspecified
365.21 Intermittent angle-closure glaucoma
365.22 Acute angle-closure glaucoma
365.23 Chronic angle-closure glaucoma
365.24 Residual stage of angle-closure glaucoma
365.42 Glaucoma associated with anomalies of iris
365.61 Glaucoma associated with pupillary block

Applicable HCPCS Level II Codes

A4305 Disposable drug delivery system, flow rate of 50 ml or greater per hour
A4306 Disposable drug delivery system, flow rate of 5 ml or less per hour
A4550 Surgical tray

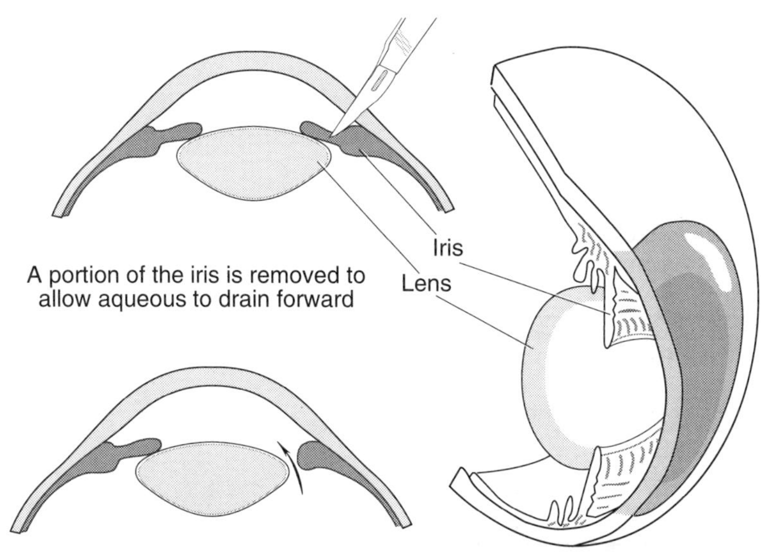

Iridectomy

66630 CPT CODE

CPT Description

Iridectomy, with corneoscleral or corneal section; sector for glaucoma (separate procedure)

Explanation

Though constantly flushed and renewed, the overall pressure of aqueous is constant in a healthy eye's anterior chamber. Too little or too much fluid can cause permanent damage. To enhance the flow of fluids in the eye, the physician makes an incision at the juncture of the cornea and sclera (the limbus). The physician then removes a wedge piece from the iris leaving what is often referred to as a keyhole pupil. This causes the intraocular pressure to fall as aqueous from behind the iris can then flow forward and drain from the eye. The physician may close the incision with sutures and may restore the intraocular pressure with an injection of water or saline. A topical antibiotic or pressure patch may be applied.

Comments

As a separate procedure, this procedure is usually an intrinsic part of a more complex service, and therefore is not reportable. However, when performed separately and for a specific purpose, it can be reported separately. For iridotomy, by photocoagulation, see 66761. This procedure is generally performed with a subconjunctival or retrobulbar injection rather than general anesthesia.

Commonly Associated ICD•9 Procedural Codes

12.39 Other iridoplasty

Follow-up Days	Assist at Surgery
30	N

Prior Approval
N

Anesthesia Code(s)
00147

Should Not Be Billed

65275 65280 65285 65800 65805 65815 65930 66020 66030 66250 66500 66600 66625 67500

Commonly Associated ICD•9 Diagnostic Codes

364.74 Adhesions and disruptions of pupillary membranes
365.20 Primary angle-closure glaucoma, unspecified
365.21 Intermittent angle-closure glaucoma
365.22 Acute angle-closure glaucoma
365.23 Chronic angle-closure glaucoma
365.24 Residual stage of angle-closure glaucoma
365.42 Glaucoma associated with anomalies of iris
365.61 Glaucoma associated with pupillary block
365.9 Unspecified glaucoma

Applicable HCPCS Level II Codes

A4305 Disposable drug delivery system, flow rate of 50 ml or greater per hour
A4306 Disposable drug delivery system, flow rate of 5 ml or less per hour
A4550 Surgical tray

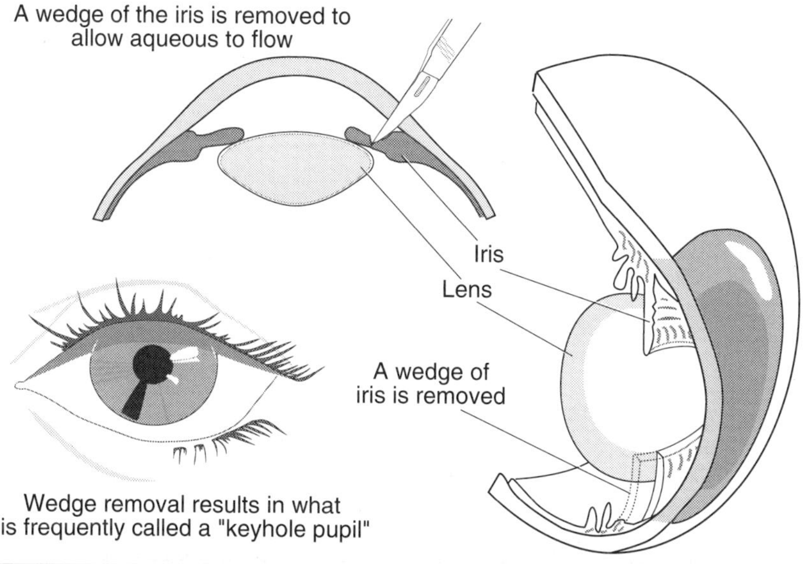

66635 CPT CODE

CPT Description

Iridectomy, with corneoscleral or corneal section; "optical" (separate procedure)

Explanation

After placing an ocular speculum in the patient's eye, the physician makes an incision at the juncture of the cornea and sclera (the limbus). The physician then trims an inner ring of iris as a means of widening an abnormally small pupil and improving vision. The physician may close the incision with sutures and may restore the intraocular pressure with an injection of water or saline. A topical antibiotic or pressure patch may be applied.

Comments

As a separate procedure, this procedure is usually an intrinsic part of a more complex service, and therefore is not reportable. However, when performed separately and for a specific purpose, it can be reported separately. For iridotomy, by photocoagulation, see 66761. This procedure is generally performed with a subconjunctival or retrobulbar injection rather than general anesthesia.

Commonly Associated ICD•9 Procedural Codes

12.39 Other iridoplasty

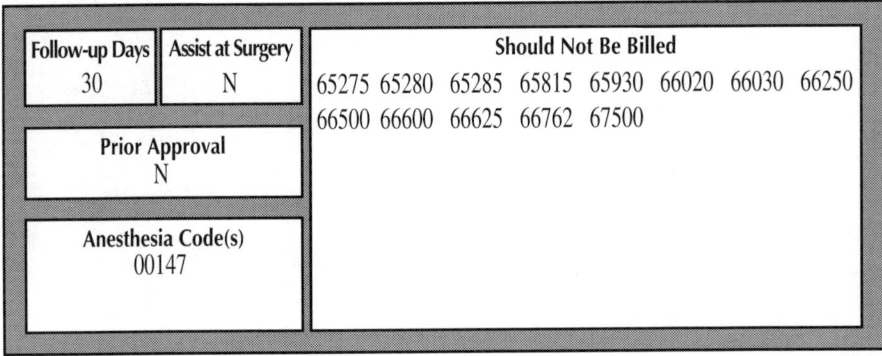

Follow-up Days	Assist at Surgery	Should Not Be Billed
30	N	65275 65280 65285 65815 65930 66020 66030 66250 66500 66600 66625 66762 67500

Prior Approval
N

Anesthesia Code(s)
00147

Commonly Associated ICD•9 Diagnostic Codes

379.40 Abnormal pupillary function, unspecified
379.42 Miosis (persistent), not due to miotics
379.45 Argyll robertson pupil, atypical

Applicable HCPCS Level II Codes

A4305 Disposable drug delivery system, flow rate of 50 ml or greater per hour
A4306 Disposable drug delivery system, flow rate of 5 ml or less per hour
A4550 Surgical tray

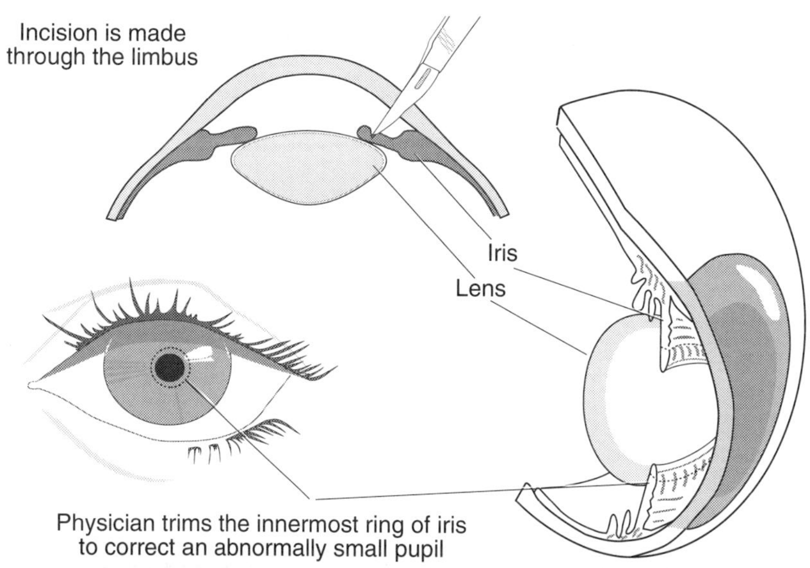

IRIDECTOMY

CPT Description

66680 Repair of iris, ciliary body (as for iridodialysis)

66682 Suture of iris, ciliary body (separate procedure) with retrieval of suture through small incision (eg, McCannel suture)

Explanation

After placing an ocular speculum in the patient's eye, the physician makes an incision at the juncture of the cornea and sclera (the limbus) to approach and repair a trauma-caused tear of the iris from from the ciliary body. The wedge shaped tear is affixed to the ciliary body with dissolving sutures, or with stitches that can be removed through an incision prepared for that retrieval. This procedure includes the later removal of the McCannel suture. The physician may close the incision with sutures and may restore the intraocular pressure with an injection of water or saline. A topical antibiotic or pressure patch may be applied.

Comments

For reposition or resection of uveal tissue with perforating wound of cornea or sclera, see 65285. As a separate procedure, 66682 is usually an intrinsic part of a more complex service, and therefore is not reportable. However, when performed separately and for a specific purpose, it can be reported separately. This procedure is generally performed with a subconjunctival or retrobulbar injection rather than general anesthesia.

Commonly Associated ICD•9 Procedural Codes

12.39 Other iridoplasty

Follow-up Days	Assist at Surgery
30	N

Prior Approval
N

Anesthesia Code(s)
00140

Should Not Be Billed
65275 65280 65285 65800 65805 65815 65930 66020 66030 66250 66500 66600 66682 66770 67500

Commonly Associated ICD•9 Diagnostic Codes

364.8 Other disorders of iris and ciliary body
871.1 Ocular laceration with prolapse or exposure of intraocular tissue

Applicable HCPCS Level II Codes

A4305 Disposable drug delivery system, flow rate of 50 ml or greater per hour
A4306 Disposable drug delivery system, flow rate of 5 ml or less per hour
A4550 Surgical tray

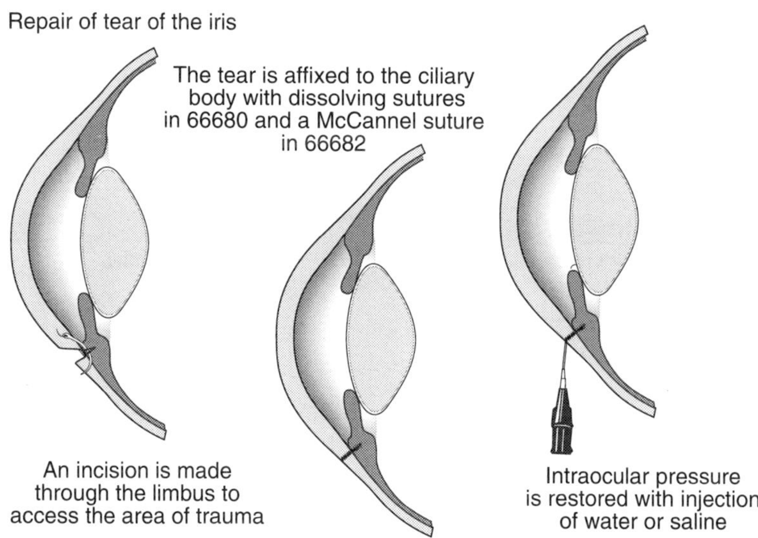

CPT Description

66700 Ciliary body destruction; diathermy

66710 cyclophotocoagulation

Explanation

The ciliary body supplies the anterior chamber with aqueous. In cases where high intraocular pressure cannot otherwise be controlled, portions of the ciliary body are destroyed to reduce the production of aqueous. The physician makes an incision in the conjunctiva and sclera in the pars plana opposite from the site to be treated. The physician uses a heat probe (diathermy) or laser (cyclophotocoagulation) to burn holes in the ciliary body. The physician closes the incision with layered sutures and may restore the intraocular pressure with an anterior and/or posterior injection. A topical antibiotic or pressure patch may be applied.

Comments

For cryotherapy, see 66720. This procedure is generally performed with topical anesthetic or subconjunctival injection rather than general anesthesia.

Commonly Associated ICD•9 Procedural Codes

12.71 Cyclodiathermy

12.74 Diminution of ciliary body, not otherwise specified

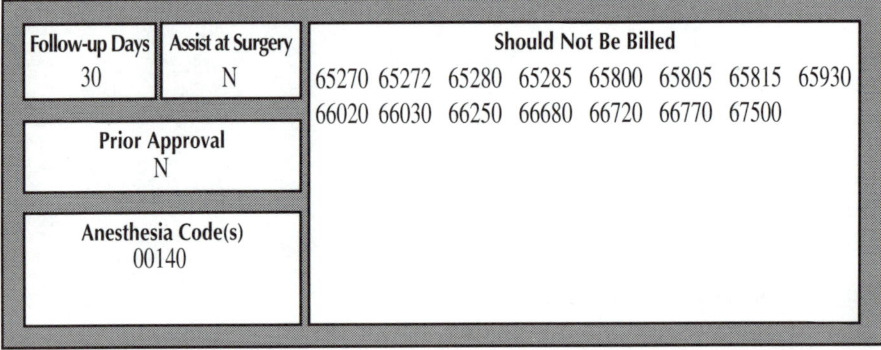

Follow-up Days	Assist at Surgery
30	N

Prior Approval
N

Anesthesia Code(s)
00140

Should Not Be Billed
65270 65272 65280 65285 65800 65805 65815 65930
66020 66030 66250 66680 66720 66770 67500

Commonly Associated ICD•9 Diagnostic Codes

365.11 Primary open angle glaucoma
365.23 Chronic angle-closure glaucoma
365.41 Glaucoma associated with chamber angle anomalies
365.63 Glaucoma associated with vascular disorders

Applicable HCPCS Level II Codes

A4305 Disposable drug delivery system, flow rate of 50 ml or greater per hour
A4306 Disposable drug delivery system, flow rate of 5 ml or less per hour
A4550 Surgical tray

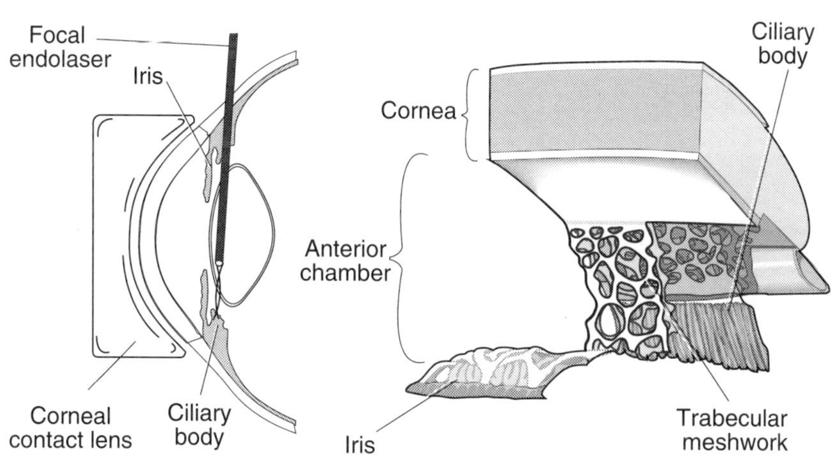

Physician uses a heat probe (66700) or laser (66710) to destroy a portion of the ciliary body

Ciliary Body Destruction

66720 CPT CODE

CPT Description

Ciliary body destruction; cryotherapy

Explanation

The ciliary body supplies the anterior chamber with aqueous. In cases where high intraocular pressure cannot otherwise be controlled, portions of the ciliary body are destroyed to reduce the production of aqueous. The physician applies a freezing probe to the sclera over the ciliary body with the purpose of destroying the ciliary process. This is especially useful in aphakic patients.

Comments

For ciliary body destruction by diathermy or cyclophotocoagulation, see 66700 and 66710. For cyclodialysis, see 66740. This procedure is generally performed with a subconjunctival injection or topical anesthetic rather than general anesthesia.

Commonly Associated ICD•9 Procedural Codes

12.72 Cyclocryotherapy

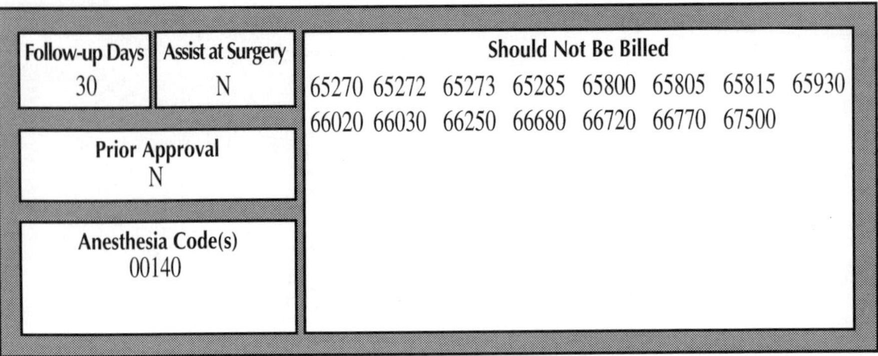

Follow-up Days	Assist at Surgery	Should Not Be Billed
30	N	65270 65272 65273 65285 65800 65805 65815 65930 66020 66030 66250 66680 66720 66770 67500

Prior Approval
N

Anesthesia Code(s)
00140

Commonly Associated ICD•9 Diagnostic Codes

360.42 Blind hypertensive eye
365.15 Residual stage of open angle glaucoma
365.63 Glaucoma associated with vascular disorders

Applicable HCPCS Level II Codes

A4305 Disposable drug delivery system, flow rate of 50 ml or greater per hour
A4306 Disposable drug delivery system, flow rate of 5 ml or less per hour
A4550 Surgical tray

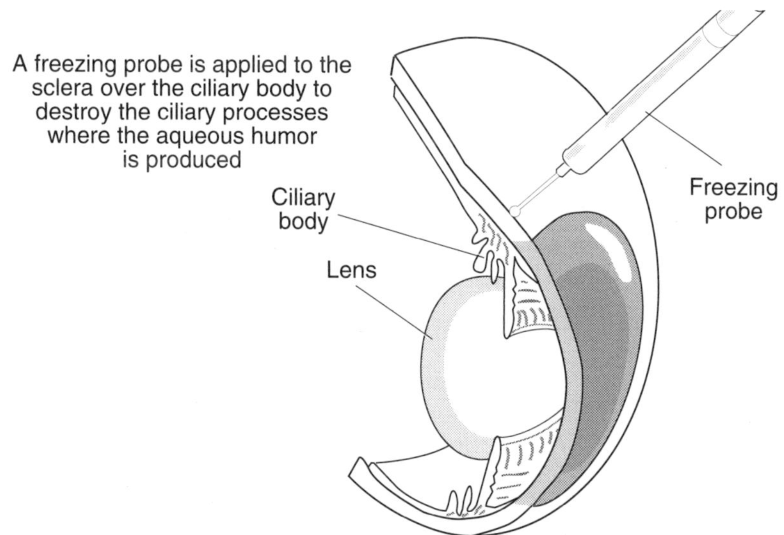

CILIARY BODY DESTRUCTION

66740 CPT CODE

CPT Description

Ciliary body destruction; cyclodialysis

Explanation

The ciliary body supplies the anterior chamber with aqueous. In cases where high intraocular pressure cannot otherwise be controlled, portions of the ciliary body are destroyed to reduce the production of aqueous. The physician makes an incision in the conjunctiva and sclera in the pars plana adjacent to the portion of ciliary body to be treated. The physician passes a spatula through the incision and into the suprachoroidal space of the anterior chamber. The spatula separates the ciliary body from the scleral spur. This may result in a lowering of intraocular pressure either by a decrease in aqueous humor formation from the now detached ciliary body or or by increasing uveovascular scleral outflow of aqueous. The physician closes the incision with layered sutures and may restore the intraocular pressure with an anterior and/or posterior injection. A topical antibiotic or pressure patch may be applied.

Comments

For ciliary body destruction by diathermy or cyclophotocoagulation, see 66700 and 66710. For cryotherapy, see 66720. This procedure is generally performed with a subconjunctival or retrobulbar injection rather than general anesthesia.

Commonly Associated ICD•9 Procedural Codes

12.55 Cyclodialysis

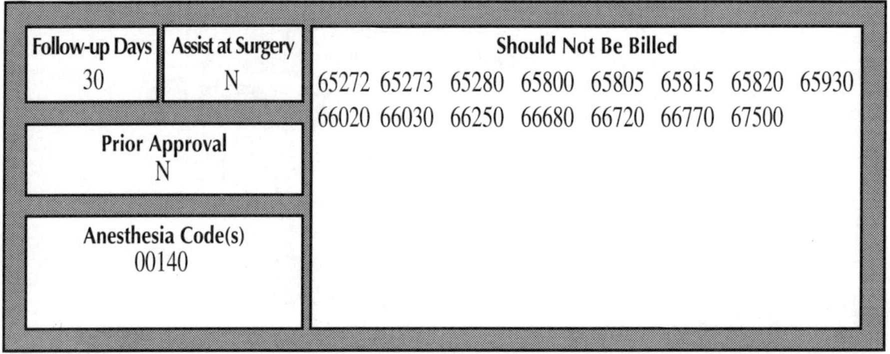

Follow-up Days	Assist at Surgery
30	N

Prior Approval
N

Anesthesia Code(s)
00140

Should Not Be Billed
65272 65273 65280 65800 65805 65815 65820 65930
66020 66030 66250 66680 66720 66770 67500

Commonly Associated ICD•9 Diagnostic Codes

364.41 Hyphema of iris and ciliary body
364.42 Rubeosis iridis
365.44 Glaucoma associated with systemic syndromes
365.42 Glaucoma associated with anomalies of iris
365.43 Glaucoma associated with other anterior segment anomalies

Applicable HCPCS Level II Codes

A4305 Disposable drug delivery system, flow rate of 50 ml or greater per hour
A4306 Disposable drug delivery system, flow rate of 5 ml or less per hour
A4550 Surgical tray

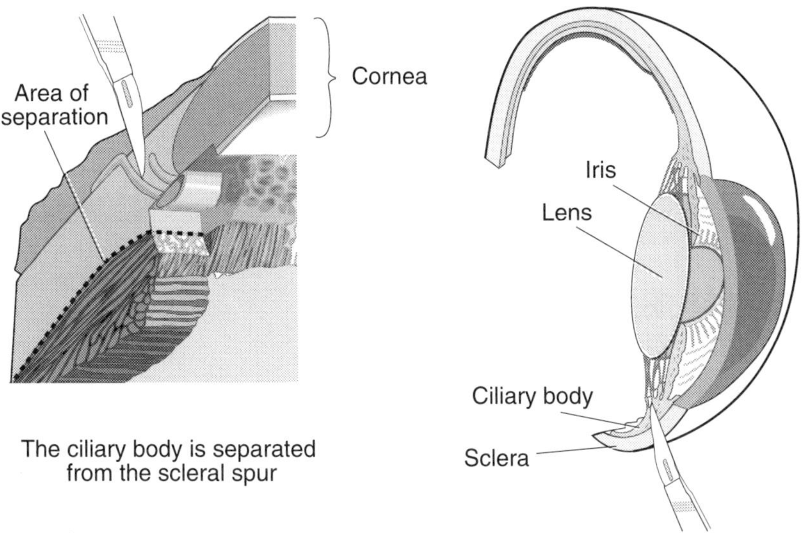

The ciliary body is separated from the scleral spur

66761 CPT CODE

CPT Description

Iridotomy/iridectomy by laser surgery (eg, for glaucoma) (one or more sessions)

Explanation

After applying a topical anesthetic, the physician places a special contact lens on the eye of the patient. The argon or YAG laser is focused on the iris and multiple short bursts of laser light create holes in the iris. This procedure allows fluids in the eye to pass from behind the iris through the openings into the space between the iris and the cornea (the anterior chamber). This lowers intraocular pressure.

Comments

For iridoplasty, use 66762. This procedure is generally performed with a topical anesthetic rather than general anesthesia.

Commonly Associated ICD•9 Procedural Codes

12.59 Other facilitation of intraocular circulation

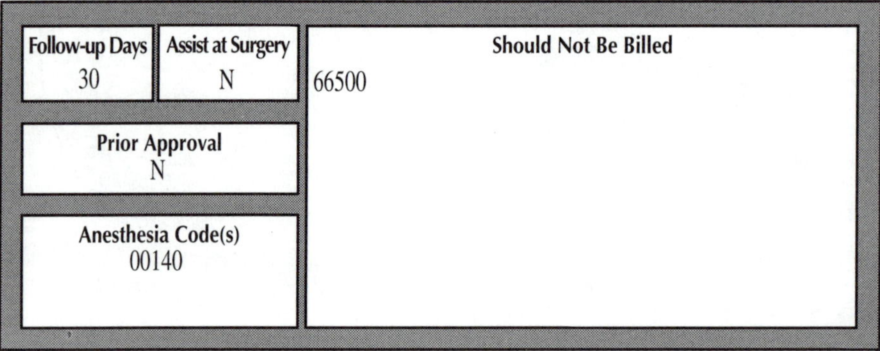

Follow-up Days	Assist at Surgery	Should Not Be Billed
30	N	66500

Prior Approval
N

Anesthesia Code(s)
00140

Commonly Associated ICD•9 Diagnostic Codes

365.20 Primary angle-closure glaucoma, unspecified
365.21 Intermittent angle-closure glaucoma
365.22 Acute angle-closure glaucoma
365.23 Chronic angle-closure glaucoma
365.24 Residual stage of angle-closure glaucoma
365.42 Glaucoma associated with anomalies of iris
365.43 Glaucoma associated with other anterior segment anomalies

Applicable HCPCS Level II Codes

A4305 Disposable drug delivery system, flow rate of 50 ml or greater per hour
A4306 Disposable drug delivery system, flow rate of 5 ml or less per hour
A4550 Surgical tray

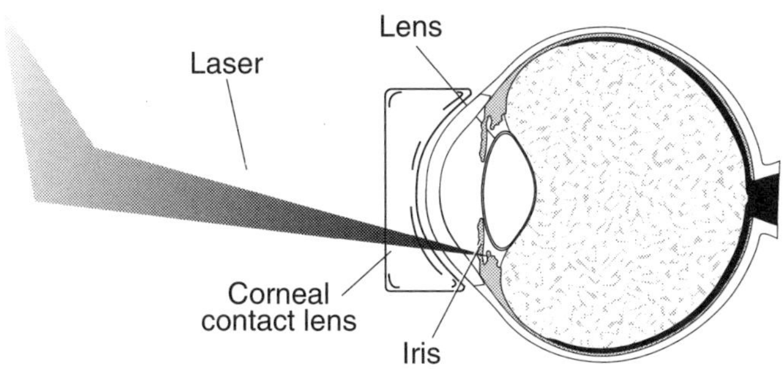

CPT Description

Iridoplasty by photocoagulation (one or more sessions) (eg, for improvement of vision, for widening of anterior chamber angle)

Explanation

The physician places a special contact lens on the eye of the patient and uses multiple bursts of light from an argon laser to create an additional hole in the iris.

Comments

More than one treatment is usually required in this therapy, but the single code includes multiple sessions. This procedure is generally performed with a topical anesthetic rather than general anesthesia.

Commonly Associated ICD•9 Procedural Codes

12.39 Other iridoplasty

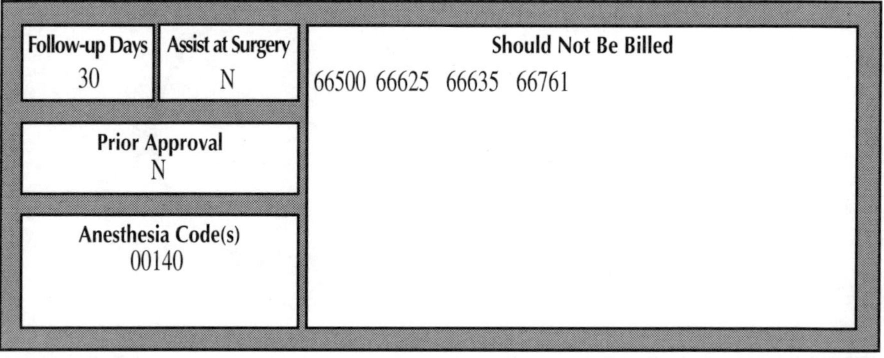

Follow-up Days	Assist at Surgery	Should Not Be Billed
30	N	66500 66625 66635 66761

Prior Approval
N

Anesthesia Code(s)
00140

Commonly Associated ICD•9 Diagnostic Codes

364.76 Iridodialysis
379.42 Miosis (persistent), not due to miotics
871.1 Ocular laceration with prolapse or exposure of intraocular tissue

Applicable HCPCS Level II Codes

A4305 Disposable drug delivery system, flow rate of 50 ml or greater per hour
A4306 Disposable drug delivery system, flow rate of 5 ml or less per hour
A4550 Surgical tray

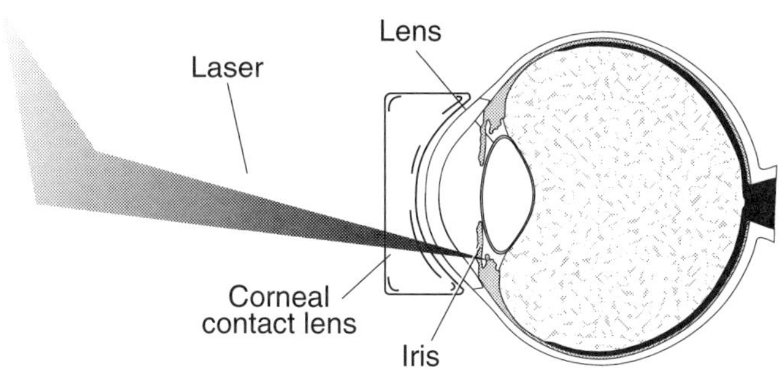

66770 CPT CODE

CPT Description

Destruction of cyst or lesion iris or ciliary body (nonexcisional procedure)

Explanation

The physician places a special contact lens on the eye of the patient. The YAG or Argon laser is focused on the cyst or lesion and multiple short bursts of light destroy the abnormal tissue.

Comments

For excision of lesion, use 66600 or 66605. For the removal of an epithelial downgrowth, see 65900. This procedure is generally performed with a topical anesthetic rather than general anesthesia.

Commonly Associated ICD•9 Procedural Codes

12.41 Destruction of lesion of iris, nonexcisional
12.43 Destruction of lesion of ciliary body, nonexcisional

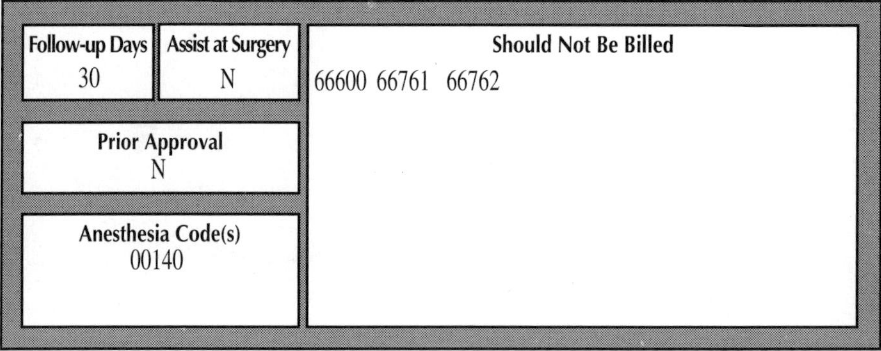

Follow-up Days	Assist at Surgery	Should Not Be Billed
30	N	66600 66761 66762

Prior Approval
N

Anesthesia Code(s)
00140

Commonly Associated ICD•9 Diagnostic Codes

224.0 Benign neoplasm of eyeball, except conjunctiva, cornea, retina, and choroid
364.55 Miotic cysts of pupillary margin
364.60 Idiopathic cysts of iris and ciliary body
364.61 Implantation cysts of iris and ciliary body
364.62 Exudative cysts of iris or anterior chamber
364.64 Exudative cyst of pars plana

Applicable HCPCS Level II Codes

A4305 Disposable drug delivery system, flow rate of 50 ml or greater per hour
A4306 Disposable drug delivery system, flow rate of 5 ml or less per hour
A4550 Surgical tray

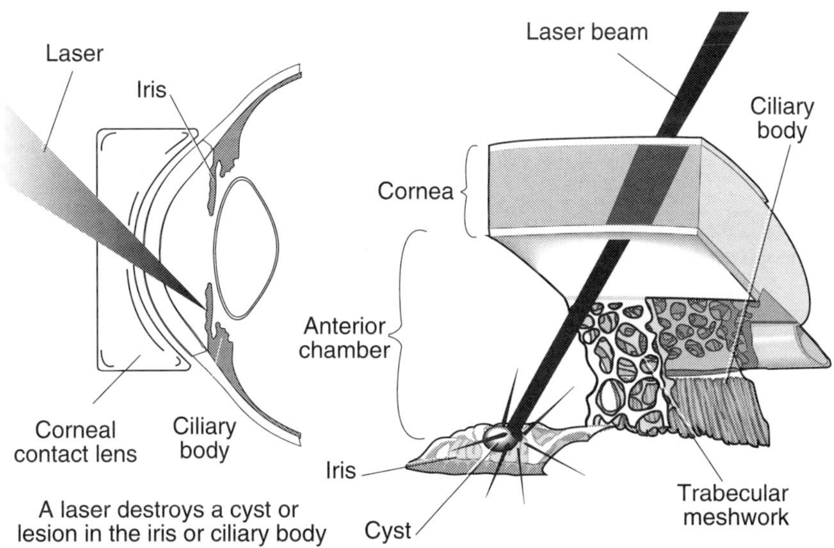

A laser destroys a cyst or lesion in the iris or ciliary body

Destruction of Cyst or Lesion

66820 CPT CODE

CPT Description

Discission of secondary membraneous cataract (opacified posterior lens capsule and/or anterior hyaloid; stab incision technique (Ziegler or Wheeler knife)

Explanation

The patient initially had extracapsular cataract surgery in which the posterior shell of the lens was not removed from the eye. But the capsule and/or the membrane adjacent to it (the anterior hyaloid) has since become opaque and must be opened in this new surgery. After placing an ocular speculum in the patient's eye, the pupil is dilated. The physician inserts a small needle, a Ziegler or Wheeler knife or special scissors into the corneal-scleral juncture (the limbus) and advances it to the edge of the capsule and through to the membrane, cutting a flap in the opaque membrane in the field of vision. The physician maneuvers the instrument around any artificial lens. No tissue is removed from the eye; the flap simply opens a window of vision. The physician may close the incision with sutures and may restore the intraocular pressure with an injection of water or saline. A topical antibiotic or pressure patch may be applied.

Comments

Code with caution. Most secondary membranous cataracts are today treated with laser surgery, not knife discission. Also, if tissue is removed, use 66830. This procedure is generally performed with a retrobulbar injection rather than general anesthesia.

Commonly Associated ICD•9 Procedural Codes

13.66 Mechanical fragmentation of secondary membrane (after cataract)

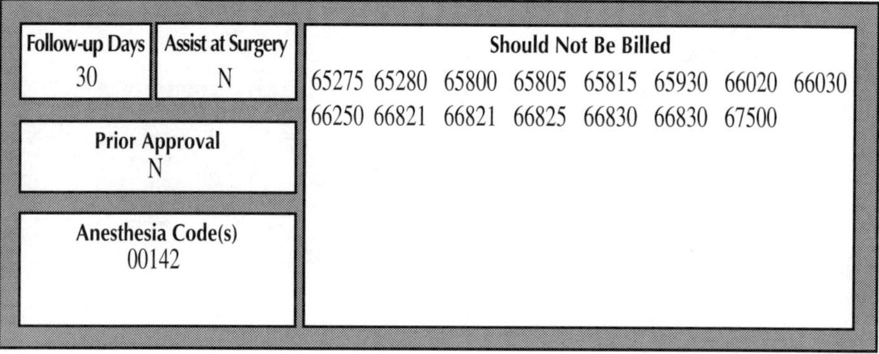

Follow-up Days	Assist at Surgery
30	N

Prior Approval
N

Anesthesia Code(s)
00142

Should Not Be Billed

65275 65280 65800 65805 65815 65930 66020 66030
66250 66821 66821 66825 66830 66830 67500

Commonly Associated ICD•9 Diagnostic Codes

366.50 After-cataract, unspecified
366.51 Soemmering's ring
366.52 Other after-cataract, not obscuring vision
366.53 After-cataract, obscuring vision
996.53 Mechanical complication of ocular lens prosthesis

Applicable HCPCS Level II Codes

A4305 Disposable drug delivery system, flow rate of 50 ml or greater per hour
A4306 Disposable drug delivery system, flow rate of 5 ml or less per hour
A4550 Surgical tray

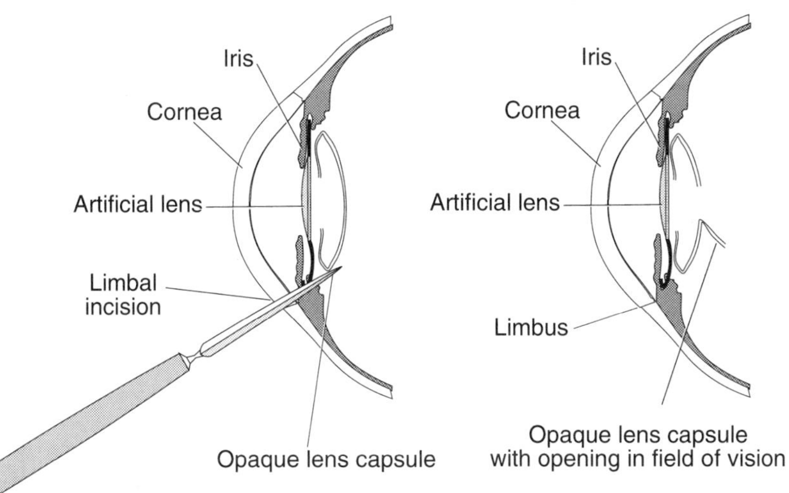

66821 CPT CODE

CPT Description

Discission of secondary membraneous cataract (opacified posterior lens capsule and/or anterior hyaloid; laser surgery (eg, YAG laser) (one or more stages)

Explanation

The patient initially had extracapsular cataract surgery in which the posterior shell of the lens was not removed from the eye. But the capsule and/or the membrane adjacent to it (the anterior hyaloid) has since become opaque and must be destroyed in this new surgery. After a topical anesthetic is applied to the eye, the pupil is dilated. A number of YAG laser shots are focused to a point on the capsule, cutting it. Bursts from the YAG open a flap in the capsule, resulting in immediate improvement in vision. Multiple sessions may be needed to create an adequate opening in the lens capsule.

Comments

If multiple sessions are needed to create an adequate opening in the lens capsule, report together under this code once. This procedure is generally performed with a topical anesthetic or retrobulbar injection rather than general anesthesia.

Commonly Associated ICD•9 Procedural Codes

13.64 Discission of secondary membrane (after cataract)

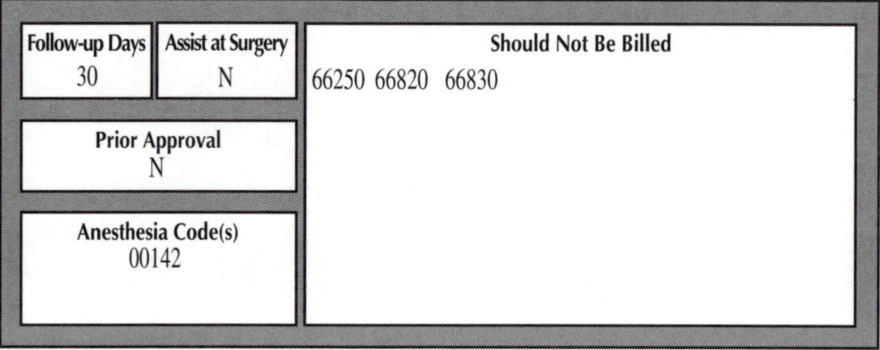

Follow-up Days	Assist at Surgery	Should Not Be Billed
30	N	66250 66820 66830

Prior Approval
N

Anesthesia Code(s)
00142

Commonly Associated ICD•9 Diagnostic Codes

366.50 After-cataract, unspecified
366.51 Soemmering's ring
366.52 Other after-cataract, not obscuring vision
366.53 After-cataract, obscuring vision
996.53 Mechanical complication of ocular lens prosthesis

Applicable HCPCS Level II Codes

A4305 Disposable drug delivery system, flow rate of 50 ml or greater per hour
A4306 Disposable drug delivery system, flow rate of 5 ml or less per hour
A4550 Surgical tray

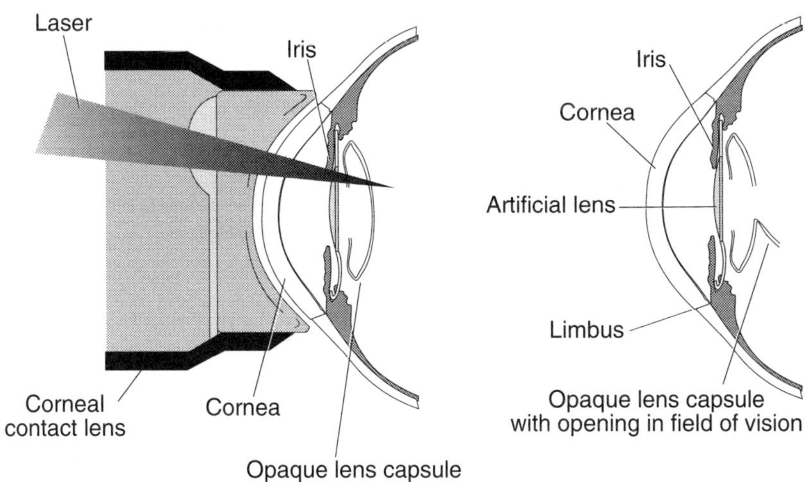

66825 CPT CODE

CPT Description

Repositioning of intraocular lens prosthesis, requiring an incision (separate procedure)

Explanation

The physician inserts a lid speculum between the patient's eyelids and the eye is secured by a suture. The physician cuts an opening at the juncture of the cornea and sclera (limbus) to access the artificial lens. The physician adjusts the artificial lens so that the attachments (haptics) of the implant are secured. The physician may close the incision with sutures and may restore the intraocular pressure with an injection of water or saline. A topical antibiotic or pressure patch may be applied.

Comments

For removal of an intraocular lens from the anterior segment, use 65920. For removal of a posterior lens, use 67121. If the lens is replaced in the anterior segment, use 66986. This separate procedure, by definition, is usually a component of a larger procedure. However, when the IOL is repositioned as the sole procedure, it should be reported using 66825. This procedure is generally performed with a retrobulbar injection rather than general anesthesia.

Commonly Associated ICD•9 Procedural Codes

13.9 Other operations on lens

Follow-up Days	Assist at Surgery	Should Not Be Billed
30	N	65275 65280 65280 65285 65800 65805 65815 65930 66020 66030 66250 66985 66986 67500
Prior Approval		
N		
Anesthesia Code(s)		
00142		

Commonly Associated ICD•9 Diagnostic Codes

368.15 Other visual distortions and entoptic phenomena
368.3 Other disorders of binocular vision
379.33 Anterior dislocation of lens
379.34 Posterior dislocation of lens
921.3 Contusion of eyeball
996.53 Mechanical complication of ocular lens prosthesis

Applicable HCPCS Level II Codes

A4305 Disposable drug delivery system, flow rate of 50 ml or greater per hour
A4306 Disposable drug delivery system, flow rate of 5 ml or less per hour
A4550 Surgical tray

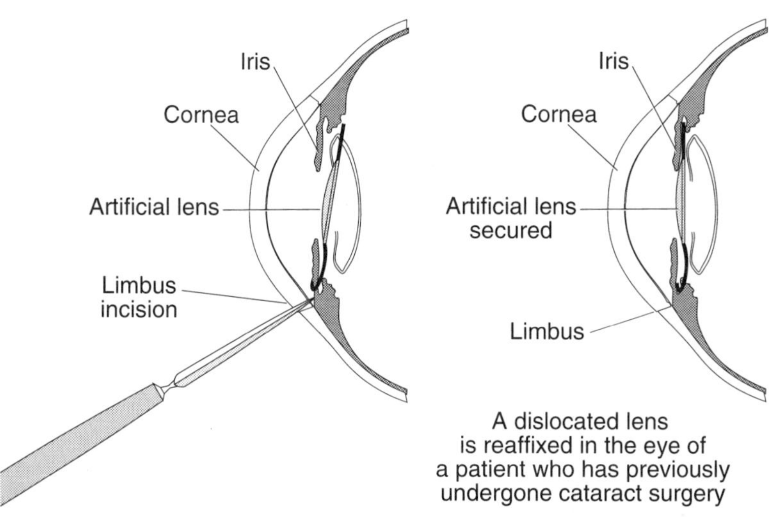

A dislocated lens is reaffixed in the eye of a patient who has previously undergone cataract surgery

66830 CPT CODE

CPT Description

Removal of secondary membranous cataract (opacified posterior lens capsule and/or anterior hyaloid) with corneo-scleral section, with or without iridectomy (iridocapsulotomy, iridocapsulectomy)

Explanation

The patient initially had extracapsular cataract surgery, in which the posterior shell of the lens was not removed from the eye. But the capsule and/or the membrane adjacent to it (the anterior hyaloid) has since become opaque and must be removed in this new surgery. The physician inserts an ocular speculum into the patient's orbit, and makes an incision at the juncture of the cornea and sclera (the limbus). A small cutting needle and suction device (an irrigating cystotome) is inserted to chip away the posterior lens capsule. In some cases, the iris must be cut ora piece of iris removed to access the lens capsule. The adjacent membrane (the anterior hyaloid) may also removed. The physician irrigates the area during aspiration. The physician may close the incision with sutures and may restore the intraocular pressure with an injection of water or saline. A topical antibiotic or pressure patch may be applied.

Comments

If no tissue is removed, use 66820. Injection is included in any cataract surgery. The use of viscoelastic agents, enzymatic zonulysis, and other pharmacologic agents as well as subconjunctival or sub-Tenon injections are included in this code. This procedure is generally performed with a retrobulbar injection rather than general anesthesia.

Commonly Associated ICD•9 Procedural Codes

13.65 Excision of secondary membrane (after cataract)

Follow-up Days	Assist at Surgery
30	N

Prior Approval
N

Anesthesia Code(s)
00142

Should Not Be Billed

65275 65280 65800 65805 65815 65930 66020 66030
66250 66500 66500 66505 66625 66625 66630 66635
66820 66821 66825 66985 66986 67500 67515 67715
68200

Commonly Associated ICD•9 Diagnostic Codes

364.70 Adhesions of iris, unspecified
366.51 Soemmering's ring
366.52 Other after-cataract, not obscuring vision
366.53 After-cataract, obscuring vision

Applicable HCPCS Level II Codes

A4305 Disposable drug delivery system, flow rate of 50 ml or greater per hour
A4306 Disposable drug delivery system, flow rate of 5 ml or less per hour
A4550 Surgical tray

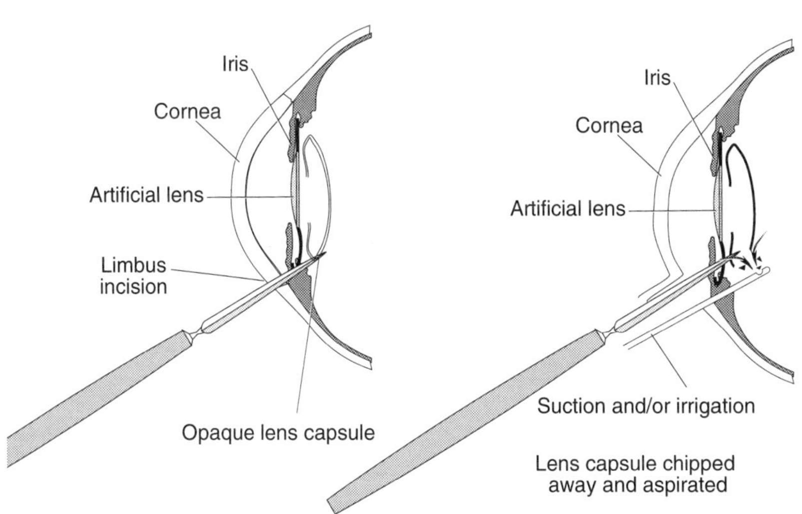

SECONDARY CATARACT REMOVAL

66840 CPT CODE

CPT Description

Removal of lens material; aspiration technique, one or more stages

Explanation

The physician makes an incision at the juncture of the cornea and sclera (the limbus). The anterior wall of the lens is incised. A probe attached to an irrigating/aspirating machine is inserted into the lens and the lens is destroyed and sucked away. The physician may close the incision with sutures and may restore the intraocular pressure with an injection of water or saline. A topical antibiotic or pressure patch may be applied.

Comments

Injection is included in any cataract surgery. The use of viscoelastic agents, enzymatic zonulysis, and other pharmacologic agents is included in this code. This procedure is generally performed with a retrobulbar injection rather than general anesthesia. This procedure is reserved for only the softest of cataracts, such as infantile cataracts, and has largely been replaced by automated irrigation and aspiration techniques.

Commonly Associated ICD•9 Procedural Codes

13.3 Extracapsular extraction of lens by simple aspiration (and irrigation) technique

Follow-up Days	Assist at Surgery
30	N

Prior Approval
N

Anesthesia Code(s)
00142

Should Not Be Billed

65275 65280 65800 65805 65815 65930 66020 66030
66250 66500 66625 66630 66635 66820 66821 66825
66985 66986 67500 67715

Commonly Associated ICD•9 Diagnostic Codes

366.00 Nonsenile cataract, unspecified
366.20 Traumatic cataract, unspecified
366.46 Cataract associated with radiation and other physical influences
366.60 Incipient senile cataract

Applicable HCPCS Level II Codes

A4305 Disposable drug delivery system, flow rate of 50 ml or greater per hour
A4306 Disposable drug delivery system, flow rate of 5 ml or less per hour
A4550 Surgical tray

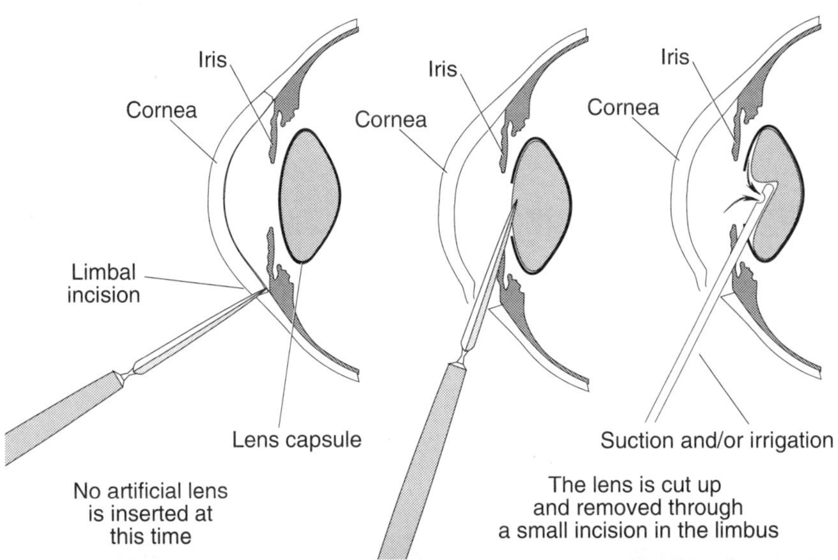

Cataract Removal

66850 CPT CODE

CPT Description

Removal of lens material; phacofragmentation technique (mechanical or ultrasonic) (eg, phacoemulsification), with aspiration

Explanation

The physician makes an incision in the cornea or the pars plana. The anterior wall of the lens is cut out. The same type of irrigating/aspirating machine used for extracapsular surgery is used for phacofragmentation, but this time the probe is a needle that vibrates 40,000 times per second (phacofragmentation), or sound waves (phacoemulsification, ultrasound) that break up the lens. The physician uses irrigation and suction to remove the once hard nucleus, now liquefied by mechanical or sound vibrations. The physician may close the incision with sutures or may design a sutureless "self-sealing" incision. The physician may restore the intraocular pressure with an injection of water or saline. A topical antibiotic or pressure patch may be applied.

Comments

Use this code for a lensectomy. Although this procedure is not mentioned as lensectomy in its official CPT description 66850, it is referenced under 67040: "For lensectomy, see 66850." If an IOL is inserted, report 66984. The use of viscoelastic agents, enzymatic zonulysis, and other pharmacologic agents as well as subconjunctival or sub-Tenon injections are included in this code. This procedure is generally performed with a local anesthetic or retrobulbar injection rather than general anesthesia.

Commonly Associated ICD•9 Procedural Codes

13.41 Phacoemulsification and aspiration of cataract

Follow-up Days	Assist at Surgery
30	N

Prior Approval
N

Anesthesia Code(s)
00142

Should Not Be Billed

65275 65280 65800 65805 65815 65930 66020 66030
66250 66500 66625 66630 66635 66820 66821 66825
66985 66986 67715

Commonly Associated ICD•9 Diagnostic Codes

366.00 Nonsenile cataract, unspecified
366.04 Nuclear nonsenile cataract
366.10 Senile cataract, unspecified
366.12 Incipient senile cataract
366.19 Other and combined forms of senile cataract
366.20 Traumatic cataract, unspecified
366.21 Localized traumatic opacities
366.22 Total traumatic cataract
366.46 Cataract associated with radiation and other physical influences

Applicable HCPCS Level II Codes

A4305 Disposable drug delivery system, flow rate of 50 ml or greater per hour
A4306 Disposable drug delivery system, flow rate of 5 ml or less per hour
A4550 Surgical tray

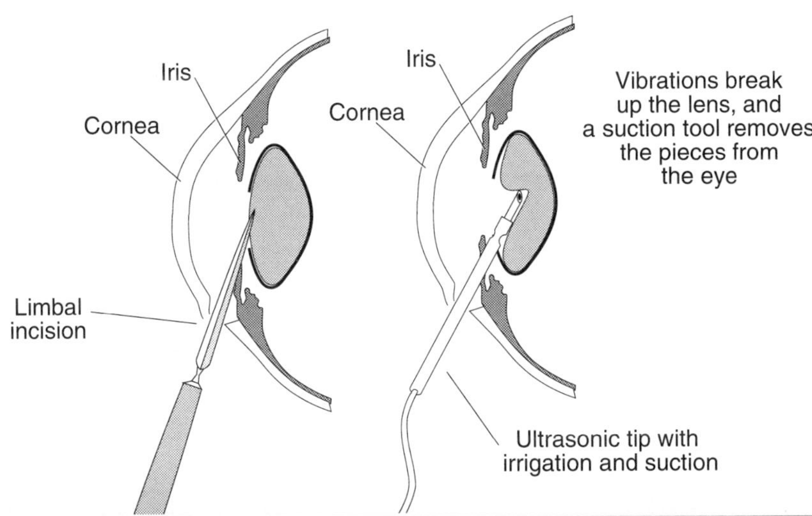

66852 CPT CODE

CPT Description

Removal of lens material; pars plana approach, with or without vitrectomy

Explanation

To remove a cataract obstructing the view of the retina during retinal surgery, or to remove a piece of natural lens retained following cataract surgery, the physician makes an incision in the conjunctiva, sclera, and choroid of the pars plana. The physician approaches the lens capsule from behind. If the entire lens is being removed, the wall of the posterior lens capsule is removed and a small suction device is inserted into the lens. The lens material is sucked out. The physician irrigates the area during aspiration. If a retained portion of the lens is removed, a portion of the clear gel in the back of the eye may be removed as well (vitrectomy). The incision is closed with layered sutures. The physician may restore anterior or posterior intraocular pressure with an injection of water or saline. A topical antibiotic or pressure patch may be applied.

Comments

Viscoelastic agents, enzymatic zonulysis, and other pharmacologic agents as well as subconjunctival or sub-Tenon injections are included in this code. This procedure is generally performed with a retrobulbar injection rather than general anesthesia.

Commonly Associated ICD•9 Procedural Codes

13.42 Mechanical phacofragmentation and aspiration of cataract by posterior route
14.74 Other mechanical vitrectomy

Follow-up Days	Assist at Surgery
30	N

Prior Approval
N

Anesthesia Code(s)
00142

Should Not Be Billed

65270	65272	65273	65280	65285	65800	65805	65810
65815	65930	66020	66030	66250	66500	66625	66630
66635	66820	66821	66825	66840	66850	66985	66986
67005	67010	67015	67025	67028	67500	67715	

Commonly Associated ICD•9 Diagnostic Codes

366.00 Nonsenile cataract, unspecified
366.04 Nuclear nonsenile cataract
366.10 Senile cataract, unspecified
366.12 Incipient senile cataract
366.19 Other and combined forms of senile cataract
366.20 Traumatic cataract, unspecified
366.21 Localized traumatic opacities
366.22 Total traumatic cataract
366.46 Cataract associated with radiation and other physical influences
998.4 Foreign body accidentally left during a procedure, not elsewhere classified

Applicable HCPCS Level II Codes

A4305 Disposable drug delivery system, flow rate of 50 ml or greater per hour
A4306 Disposable drug delivery system, flow rate of 5 ml or less per hour
A4550 Surgical tray

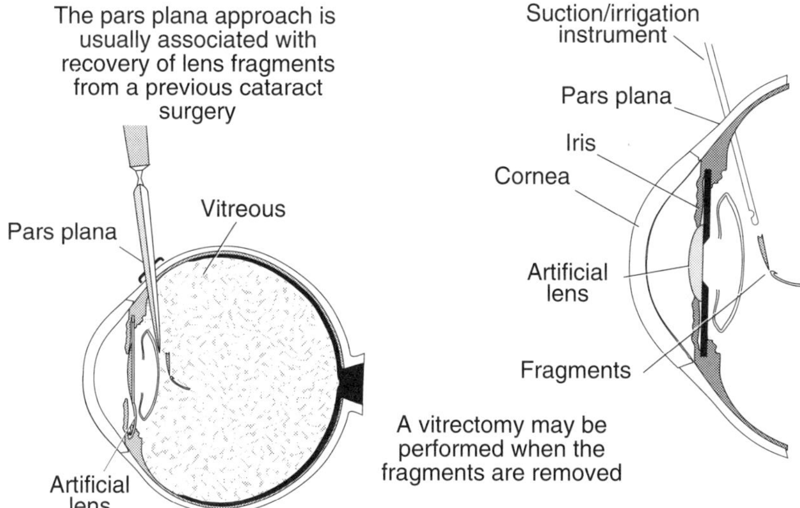

This code also reports a lensectomy performed during retinal surgery

CPT Description

66920 Removal of lens material; intracapsular

66930 for dislocated lens

Explanation

Intracapsular cataract extraction (ICCE) is when the lens and capsule are removed intact. The physician inserts an ocular speculum. An incision is made in the corneal-scleral juncture (the limbus). To enhance the flow of fluids in the eye, the physician may punch a hole in the iris before inserting a surgical instrument filled with coolant (cryoprobe) into the anterior chamber. The lens adheres to the cryoprobe as it freezes, and when the cryoprobe is removed, the lens comes with it (e.g., for 66920). The same technique is used to removed a dislocated lens (e.g., for 66930). The physician may close the incision with sutures and may restore intraocular pressure with an injection of water or saline. A topical antibiotic or pressure patch may be applied.

Comments

Viscoelastic agents, enzymatic zonulysis, and other pharmacologic agents are included in this code. This procedure is less common than extracapsular extraction. It is generally reserved for patients whose natural lenses are not secure. If the lens is removed through an ultrasound technique (phacofragmentation), use 66850; if an aspiration technique is applied, use 66840. This procedure is generally performed with a retrobulbar injection rather than general anesthesia.

Commonly Associated ICD•9 Procedural Codes

13.11 Intracapsular extraction of lens by temporal inferior route

13.19 Other intracapsular extraction of lens

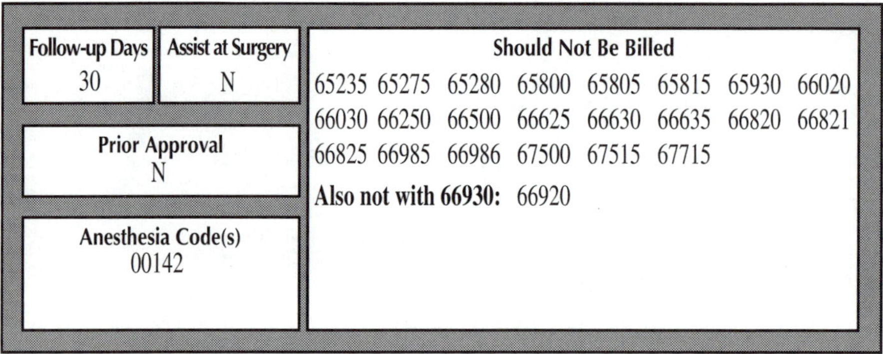

Follow-up Days	Assist at Surgery
30	N

Prior Approval
N

Anesthesia Code(s)
00142

Should Not Be Billed

65235 65275 65280 65800 65805 65815 65930 66020
66030 66250 66500 66625 66630 66635 66820 66821
66825 66985 66986 67500 67515 67715

Also not with 66930: 66920

Commonly Associated ICD•9 Diagnostic Codes

For 66920:

366.00 Nonsenile cataract, unspecified
366.04 Nuclear nonsenile cataract
366.10 Senile cataract, unspecified
366.11 Pseudoexfoliation of lens capsule
366.12 Incipient senile cataract
366.19 Other and combined forms of senile cataract
366.20 Traumatic cataract, unspecified
366.21 Localized traumatic opacities
366.22 Total traumatic cataract
366.46 Cataract associated with radiation and other physical influences

For 66930:

379.32 Subluxation of lens
379.33 Anterior dislocation of lens
379.34 Posterior dislocation of lens
379.39 Other disorders of lens

Applicable HCPCS Level II Codes

A4305 Disposable drug delivery system, flow rate of 50 ml or greater per hour
A4306 Disposable drug delivery system, flow rate of 5 ml or less per hour
A4550 Surgical tray

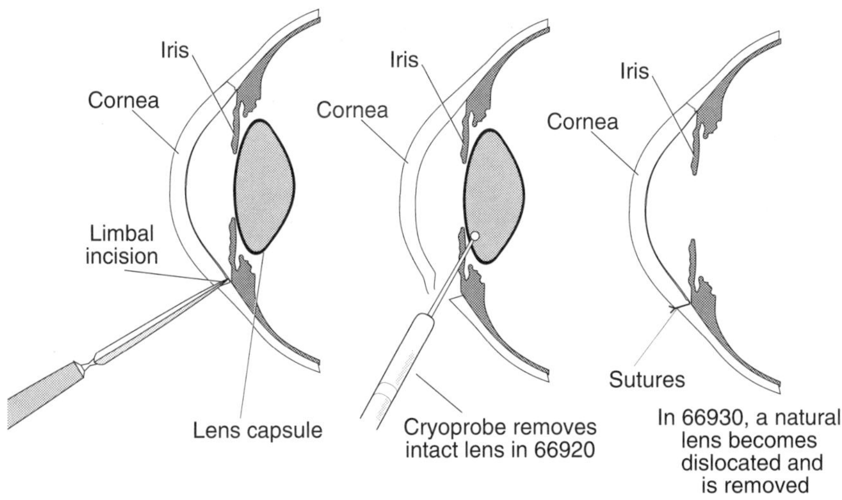

66920 is commonly called ICCE – Intracapsular cataract extraction

66940 CPT CODE

CPT Description

Removal of lens material; extracapsular (other than 66840, 66850, 66852)

Explanation

Extracapsular cataract extraction (ECCE) is when the anterior shell and the nucleus of the lens capsule are both removed, leaving the posterior shell of the lens capsule in place. The physician inserts a lid speculum between the patient's eyelids and makes an incision in the corneal-scleral juncture (the limbus). To enhance the flow of fluids in the eye, the physician may punch a hole in the iris. Using a method other than aspiration or phacofragmentation, the physician removes the lens in parts: first the anterior lens, then the inner, hard nucleus. The clear, posterior capsule remains. The physician may close the incision with sutures and may restore the intraocular pressure with an injection of water or saline. A topical antibiotic or pressure patch may be applied.

Comments

For removal of intralenticular foreign body without lens extraction, use 65235. For repair of operative wound, see 66250. Viscoelastic agents, enzymatic zonulysis, and other pharmacologic agents are included in this code. This procedure is generally performed with a retrobulbar injection rather than general anesthesia.

Commonly Associated ICD•9 Procedural Codes

13.41 Phacoemulsification and aspiration of cataract

13.42 Mechanical phacofragmentation and aspiration of cataract by posterior route

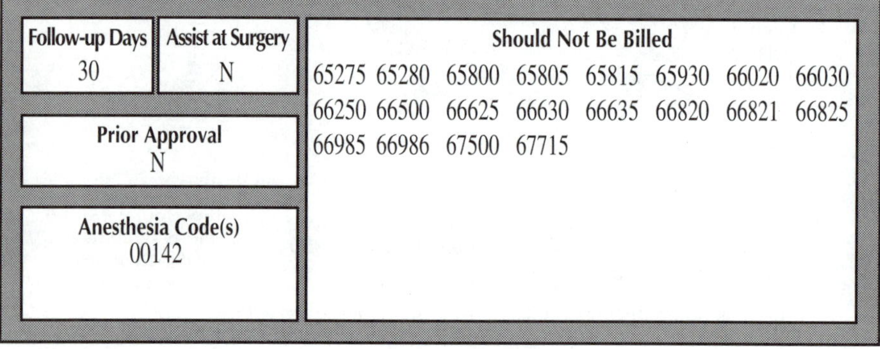

Follow-up Days	Assist at Surgery
30	N

Prior Approval
N

Anesthesia Code(s)
00142

Should Not Be Billed

65275 65280 65800 65805 65815 65930 66020 66030
66250 66500 66625 66630 66635 66820 66821 66825
66985 66986 67500 67715

Commonly Associated ICD•9 Diagnostic Codes

366.00 Nonsenile cataract, unspecified
366.04 Nuclear nonsenile cataract
366.10 Senile cataract, unspecified
366.12 Incipient senile cataract
366.19 Other and combined forms of senile cataract
366.20 Traumatic cataract, unspecified
366.21 Localized traumatic opacities
366.22 Total traumatic cataract
366.46 Cataract associated with radiation and other physical influences

Applicable HCPCS Level II Codes

A4305 Disposable drug delivery system, flow rate of 50 ml or greater per hour
A4306 Disposable drug delivery system, flow rate of 5 ml or less per hour
A4550 Surgical tray

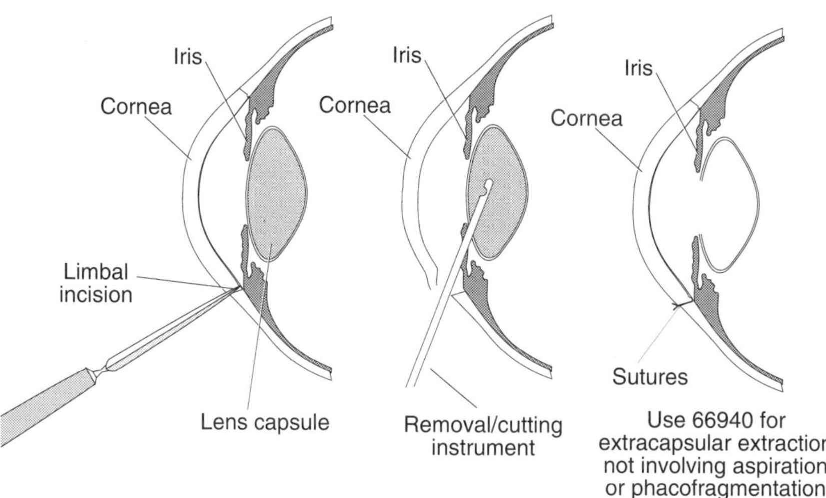

This is commonly called ECCE – Extracapsular cataract extraction

66983 CPT CODE

CPT Description

Intracapsular cataract extraction with insertion of intraocular lens prosthesis (one stage procedure)

Explanation

Intracapsular cataract extraction (ICCE) is when the lens and capsule are removed intact. The physician inserts an ocular speculum. An incision is made in the corneal-scleral juncture (the limbus). To enhance the flow of fluids in the eye, the physician may punch a hole in the iris before inserting a surgical instrument filled with coolant (cryoprobe) into the anterior chamber. The lens adheres to the cryoprobe as it freezes, and when the cryoprobe is removed, the lens comes with it. The physician injects a bubble of air into the anterior chamber to protect the cornea. The physician places an intraocular lens in the anterior chamber. The optic, or center, of the implant lies centered at the pupil and the haptics (securing attachments) of the implant are wedged in the anterior chamber, fixating the implant so it cannot move. The physician may close the incision with sutures and may restore the intraocular pressure with an injection of water or saline. A topical antibiotic or pressure patch may be applied.

Comments

For ultrasonic determination of IOL power, report 76519. This procedure is less common than extracapsular extraction. It is generally reserved for patients whose natural lenses are not secure. This procedure is generally performed with a retrobulbar injection rather than general anesthesia.

Commonly Associated ICD•9 Procedural Codes

13.11 Intracapsular extraction of lens by temporal inferior route
13.19 Other intracapsular extraction of lens

Follow-up Days	Assist at Surgery
30	N

Prior Approval
N

Anesthesia Code(s)
00142

Should Not Be Billed

65275 65280 65800 65805 65815 65930 66020 66030 66250 66500 66625 66630 66635 66820 66821 66825 66840 66850 66920 66930 66940 66985 66986 67500 67515 67715

Commonly Associated ICD•9 Diagnostic Codes

366.00 Nonsenile cataract, unspecified
366.04 Nuclear nonsenile cataract
366.10 Senile cataract, unspecified
366.12 Incipient senile cataract
366.19 Other and combined forms of senile cataract
366.20 Traumatic cataract, unspecified
366.21 Localized traumatic opacities
366.22 Total traumatic cataract
366.46 Cataract associated with radiation and other physical influences

Applicable HCPCS Level II Codes

A4305 Disposable drug delivery system, flow rate of 50 ml or greater per hour
A4306 Disposable drug delivery system, flow rate of 5 ml or less per hour
A4550 Surgical tray
V2630 Anterior chamber intraocular lens
V2631 Iris supported intraocular lens

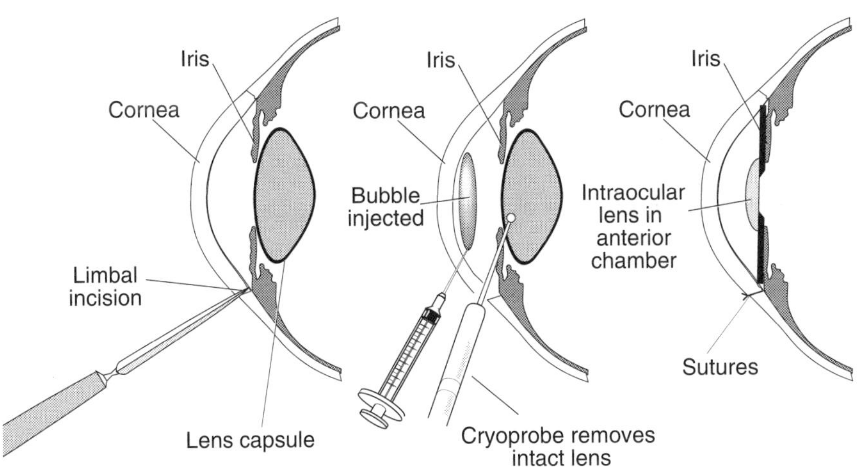

This is commonly called ICCE – Intracapsular cataract extraction

66984 CPT CODE

CPT Description

Extracapsular cataract removal with insertion of intraocular lens prosthesis (one stage procedure), manual or mechanical technique (eg, irrigation and aspiration or phacoemulsification)

Explanation

Extracapsular cataract extraction (ECCE) is when the anterior shell and the nucleus of the lens capsule are both removed, leaving the posterior shell of the lens capsule in place. The physician inserts a lid speculum between the patient's eyelids and makes an incision in the corneal-scleral juncture (the limbus). To enhance the flow of fluids in the eye, the physician may punch a hole in the iris. Using a cutting and suction or ultrasonic device, the physician removes the lens in parts: first the anterior lens, then the inner, hard nucleus. The clear, posterior capsule remains. The physician injects a bubble of air into the anterior chamber to protect the cornea. The physician then guides the intraocular implant into the eye. The haptics (securing attachments) lodge into the ciliary sulcus or the lens capsule, occupying the exact position of the original cataract. The physician may close the incision with sutures and may restore the intraocular pressure with an injection of water or saline. A topical antibiotic or pressure patch may be applied.

Comments

For intraocular lens prosthesis supplied by physician, use code 99070. For ultrasonic determination of IOL power, use 76519. This proccdure is generally performed with a retrobulbar injection rather than general anesthesia.

Commonly Associated ICD•9 Procedural Codes

13.41 Phacoemulsification and aspiration of cataract
13.43 Mechanical phacofragmentation and other aspiration of cataract

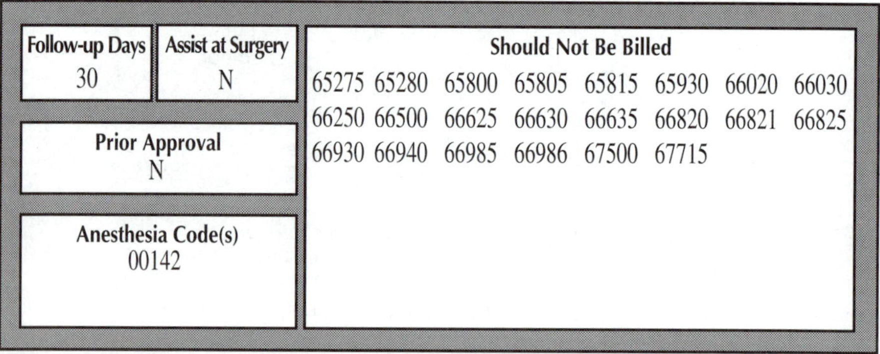

Follow-up Days	Assist at Surgery
30	N

Prior Approval
N

Anesthesia Code(s)
00142

Should Not Be Billed

65275	65280	65800	65805	65815	65930	66020	66030
66250	66500	66625	66630	66635	66820	66821	66825
66930	66940	66985	66986	67500	67715		

Commonly Associated ICD•9 Diagnostic Codes

366.00 Nonsenile cataract, unspecified
366.04 Nuclear nonsenile cataract
366.10 Senile cataract, unspecified
366.12 Incipient senile cataract
366.19 Other and combined forms of senile cataract
366.20 Traumatic cataract, unspecified
366.21 Localized traumatic opacities
366.22 Total traumatic cataract
366.46 Cataract associated with radiation and other physical influences

Applicable HCPCS Level II Codes

A4305 Disposable drug delivery system, flow rate of 50 ml or greater per hour
A4550 Surgical tray
V2630 Anterior chamber intraocular lens
V2631 Iris supported intraocular lens
V2632 Posterior chamber intraocular lens

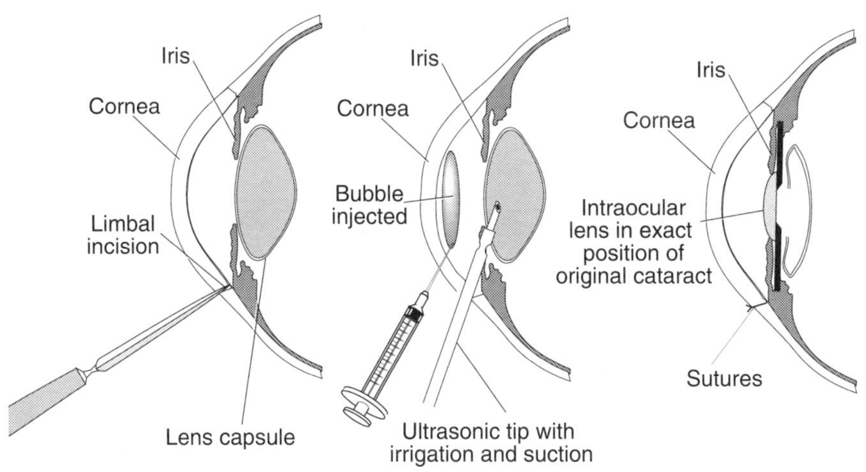

This is commonly called ECCE – extracapsular cataract extraction

66985 CPT CODE

CPT Description

Insertion of intraocular lens prosthesis (secondary implant), not associated with concurrent cataract removal

Explanation

The physician inserts an ocular speculum. An incision is made in the corneal-scleral juncture (the limbus). For an anterior lens, the physician places an intraocular lens in the fluid-filled space between the iris and cornea (the anterior chamber). The optic, or center, of the implant lies just in front of the pupil and the haptics (securing attachments) of the implant are wedged between the iris and cornea, fixating the implant so it cannot move. For a posterior lens, the physician injects a bubble of air into the anterior chamber to protect the cornea. The physician then guides the intraocular implant into the eye. The haptics lodge into the ciliary sulcus or the lens capsule. The physician may close the incision with sutures and may restore the intraocular pressure with an injection of water or saline. A topical antibiotic or pressure patch may be applied.

Comments

This procedure is usually reserved for patients who underwent traditional cataract surgery without lens implantation many years ago or who experienced a complication during initial cataract surgery which precluded lens implantation at that time. Use 66983 or 66984 for implant concurrent with cataract surgery. For intraocular lens supplied by physician, use 99070. For ultrasonic determination of intraocular lens power, use 76519. For removal of implanted material from anterior segment, use 65929. For secondary fixation (separate procedure) use 66682. This procedure is generally performed with a retrobulbar injection rather than general anesthesia.

Commonly Associated ICD•9 Procedural Codes

13.70 Insertion of pseudophakos, not otherwise specified
13.72 Secondary insertion of intraocular lens prosthesis

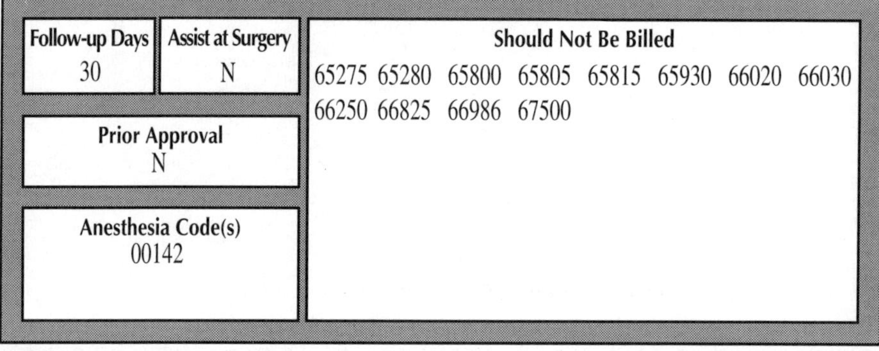

Follow-up Days	Assist at Surgery	Should Not Be Billed
30	N	65275 65280 65800 65805 65815 65930 66020 66030 66250 66825 66986 67500

Prior Approval
N

Anesthesia Code(s)
00142

Commonly Associated ICD•9 Diagnostic Codes

379.31 Aphakia
V45.6 Postsurgical states following surgery of eye and adnexa

Applicable HCPCS Level II Codes

A4305 Disposable drug delivery system, flow rate of 50 ml or greater per hour
A4550 Surgical tray
V2630 Anterior chamber intraocular lens
V2631 Iris supported intraocular lens
V2632 Posterior chamber intraocular lens

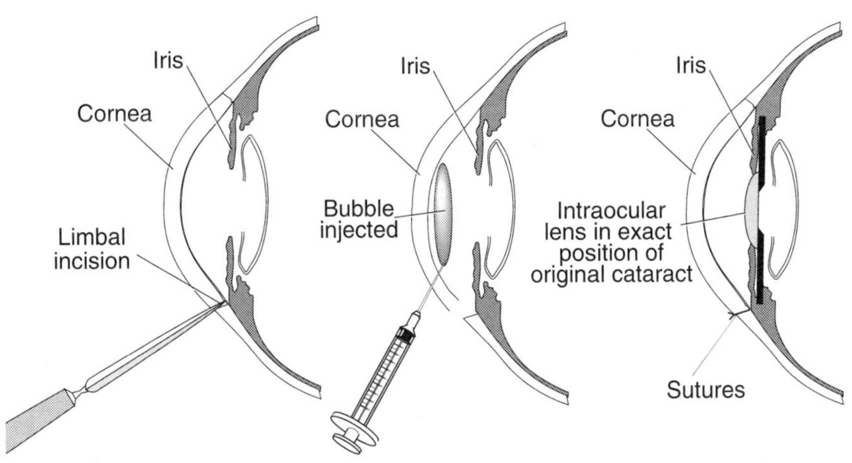

The lens is inserted in an eye that had previously undergone cataract removal

IOL Insertion

66986 CPT CODE

CPT Description

Exchange of intraocular lens

Explanation

Early models of IOL implants sometimes cause irritation in the patient's eye. They can also become dislocated. Here, the physician exchanges the problematic lens for a newer one. For anterior IOL, the physician replaces an intraocular lens in the fluid-filled space between the iris and cornea (the anterior chamber). The optic, or center, of the implant lies just in front of the pupil and the haptics (securing attachments) of the implant are lodged between the iris and cornea, fixating the implant so it cannot move. For posterior IOL, the physician injects a bubble of air into the anterior chamber through a syringe to protect the cornea. The physician then replaces the intraocular implant in the eye. The haptics lodge into the ciliary sulcus or the lens capsule. The physician may close the incision with sutures and may restore the intraocular pressure with an injection of water or saline. A topical antibiotic or pressure patch may be applied.

Comments

Use 66983 or 66984 for implant concurrent with cataract surgery. For intraocular lens supplied by physician, use 99070. For ultrasonic determination of IOL power, use 76519. This procedure is generally performed with a retrobulbar injection rather than general anesthesia.

Commonly Associated ICD•9 Procedural Codes

13.70	Insertion of pseudophakos, not otherwise specified
13.8	Removal of implanted lens

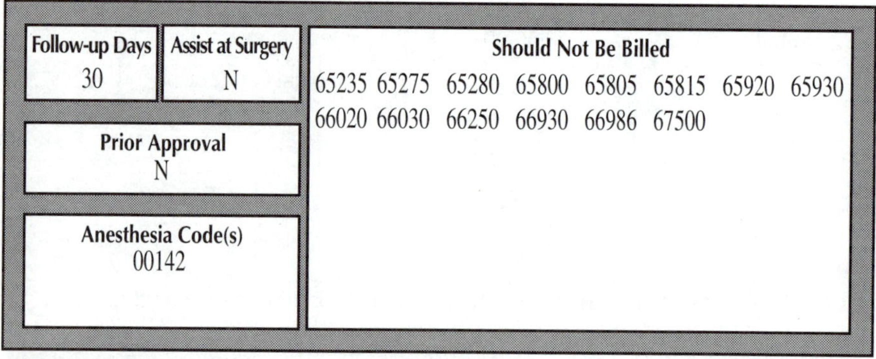

Follow-up Days	Assist at Surgery
30	N

Prior Approval
N

Anesthesia Code(s)
00142

Should Not Be Billed
65235 65275 65280 65800 65805 65815 65920 65930
66020 66030 66250 66930 66986 67500

Commonly Associated ICD•9 Diagnostic Codes

364.1 Chronic iridocyclitis
379.32 Subluxation of lens
379.33 Anterior dislocation of lens
379.34 Posterior dislocation of lens
379.39 Other disorders of lens
V43.1 Lens replaced by other means

Applicable HCPCS Level II Codes

A4550 Surgical tray
V2630 Anterior chamber intraocular lens
V2631 Iris supported intraocular lens
V2632 Posterior chamber intraocular lens
A4305 Disposable drug delivery system, flow rate of 50 ml or greater per hour

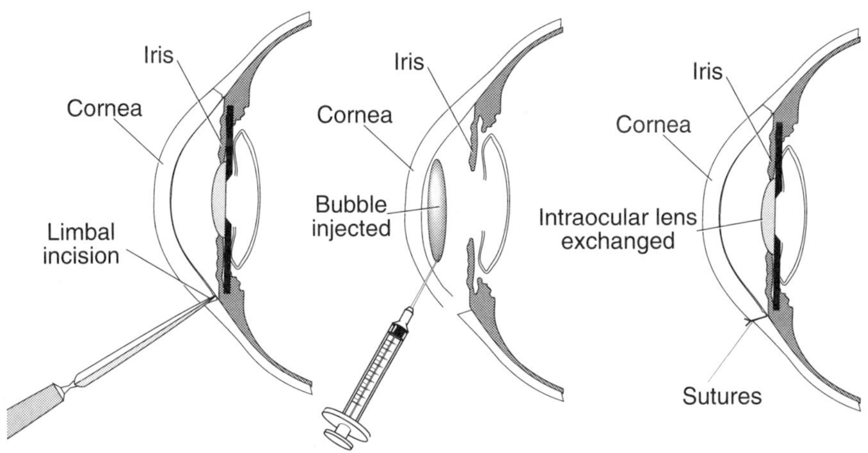

A faulty or irritating artificial lens is removed and replaced with another one

CPT Description

67005 Removal of vitreous, anterior approach (open sky technique or limbal incision); partial removal

67010 anterior approach (open sky technique or limbal incision); subtotal removal with mechanical vitrectomy

Explanation

The physician inserts a needle at the limbus or through the cornea (open sky technique) and passes the needle to the back of the anterior segment where a portion of displaced vitreous humor is aspirated (e.g., 67005). If most or all of the vitreous is extracted, mechanical tools are used (e.g., 67010). When this is done, the physician extracts the vitreous, using a mechanical cutting and suctioning process that may involve a special instrument like a rotoextractor or vitreous infusion suction cutter (VICS). In either case the aspirated vitreous is usually replaced by an injection of a vitreous substitute or aqueous. Any incision is closed with sutures.

Comments

Code with caution: this procedure is rarely performed today. For vitreous removal by paracentesis of anterior chamber, see 65810. For removal of corneovitreal adhesions, see 65880. This procedure is generally performed with a subconjunctival or retrobulbar injection rather than general anesthesia.

Commonly Associated ICD•9 Procedural Codes

14.71 Removal of vitreous, anterior approach

14.73 Mechanical vitrectomy by anterior approach

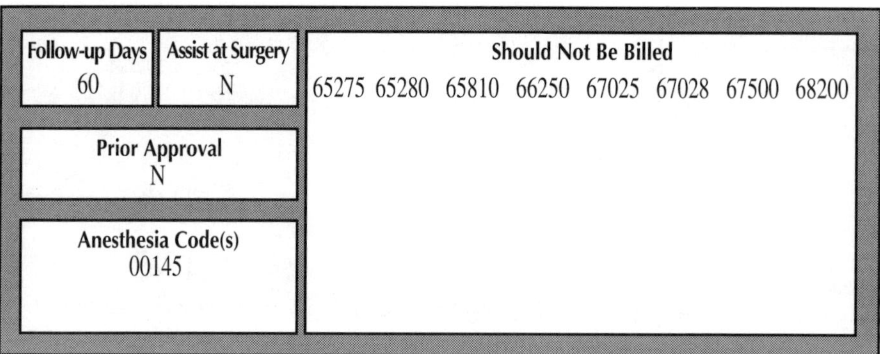

Follow-up Days	Assist at Surgery	Should Not Be Billed
60	N	65275 65280 65810 66250 67025 67028 67500 68200
Prior Approval		
N		
Anesthesia Code(s)		
00145		

Commonly Associated ICD•9 Diagnostic Codes

360.19 Other endophthalmitis
379.22 Crystalline deposits in vitreous
379.25 Vitreous membranes and strands
379.26 Vitreous prolapse
379.29 Other disorders of vitreous
998.9 Unspecified complication of procedure, not elsewhere classified

Applicable HCPCS Level II Codes

A4305 Disposable drug delivery system, flow rate of 50 ml or greater per hour
A4306 Disposable drug delivery system, flow rate of 5 ml or less per hour
A4550 Surgical tray

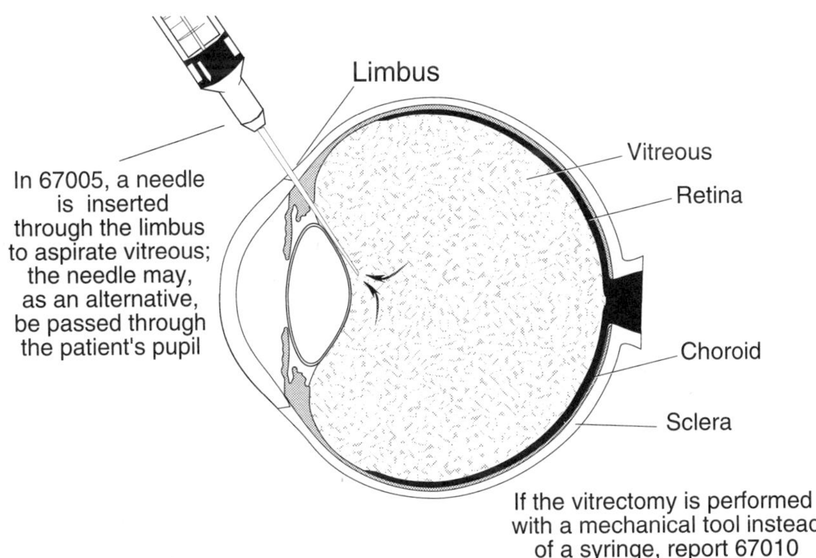

PARTIAL VITRECTOMY

67015 CPT CODE

CPT Description

Aspiration or release of vitreous, subretinal or choroidal fluid, pars plana approach (posterior sclerotomy)

Explanation

The physician inserts a needle into the posterior chamber through the pars plana to aspirate vitreous. Sometimes a posterior sclerotomy is made to release the fluid. When this is done, the physician extracts the vitreous, using a mechanical cutting and suctioning process that may involve a special instrument like a rotoextractor or vitreous infusion suction cutter (VICS). This is often called a vitreous chamber tap in operative reports. Once completed, the incision is repaired with sutures. Intraocular pressure may be adjusted with an injection. A pressure patch may be applied.

Comments

If vitreous aspirated is to be analyzed by an outside laboratory, report 99000 for the handling of the specimen. For removal of vitreous by paracentesis of anterior chamber, see 65810. For vitrectomy in retinal detachment surgery, see 67108. For unlisted procedures of the vitreous, use 67299. This procedure is generally performed with a subconjunctival or retrobulbar injection rather than general anesthesia.

Commonly Associated ICD•9 Procedural Codes

14.11 Diagnostic aspiration of vitreous

14.71 Removal of vitreous, anterior approach

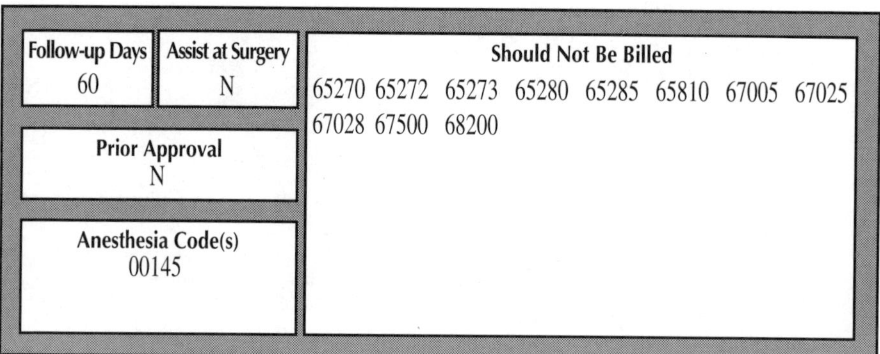

Follow-up Days	Assist at Surgery	Should Not Be Billed
60	N	65270 65272 65273 65280 65285 65810 67005 67025 67028 67500 68200
Prior Approval		
N		
Anesthesia Code(s)		
00145		

Commonly Associated ICD•9 Diagnostic Codes

362.40 Retinal layer separation, unspecified
363.6 Choroidal hemorrhage and rupture
363.7 Choroidal detachment

Applicable HCPCS Level II Codes

A4305 Disposable drug delivery system, flow rate of 50 ml or greater per hour
A4306 Disposable drug delivery system, flow rate of 5 ml or less per hour
A4550 Surgical tray

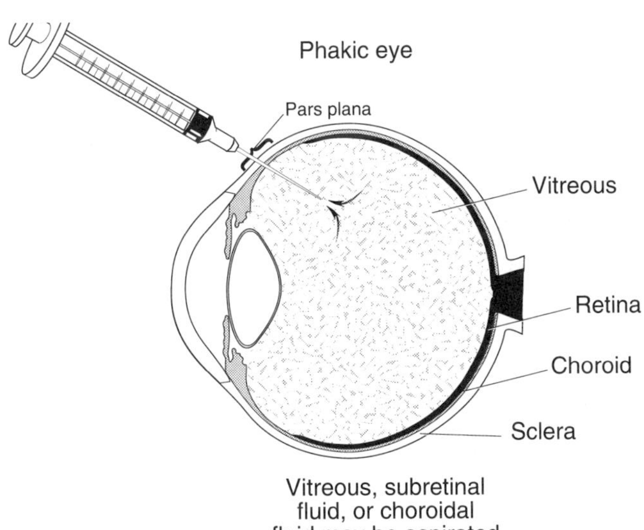

CPT Description

67025 Injection of vitreous substitute, pars plana or limbal approach, (fluid-gas exchange), with or without aspiration (separate procedure)

67028 Intravitreal injection of a pharmacologic agent (separate procedure)

Explanation

The physician inserts a sringe in the pars plana to inject a material like healon or silicone. The injection may be required to replace vitreous that has been aspirated as part of this procedure, to restore intraocular pressure lost in another manner (e.g., 67025), or to introduce medication to the posterior segment (e.g., 67028).

Comments

Both 67025 and 67028 are separate procedures, and as such, are usually components of a more complicated procedures.However, if either is performed alone and for specific purpose, it should be reported separately. If vitreous aspirated in 67025 is to be analyzed by an outside laboratory, report 99000 for the handling of the specimen. For removal of vitreous by paracentesis of anterior chamber, see 65810. For use of vitrectomy in retinal detachment surgery, see 67108. For unlisted procedures of the vitreous, use 67299. This procedure is generally performed with a retrobulbar injection rather than general anesthesia.

Commonly Associated ICD•9 Procedural Codes

14.75 Injection of vitreous substitute

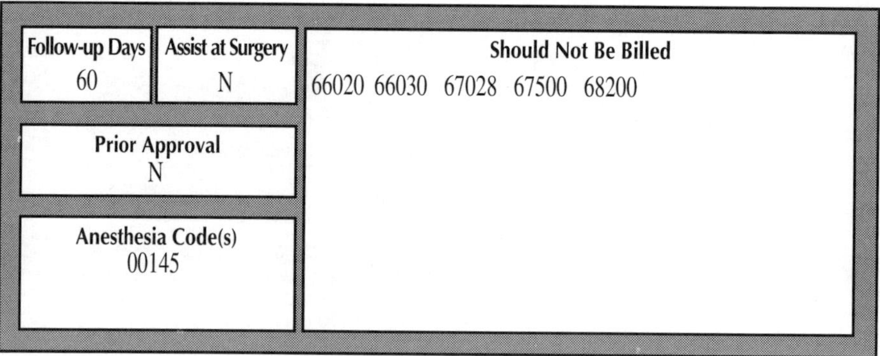

Follow-up Days	Assist at Surgery	Should Not Be Billed
60	N	66020 66030 67028 67500 68200

Prior Approval
N

Anesthesia Code(s)
00145

Commonly Associated ICD•9 Diagnostic Codes

For 67025:

361.00 Retinal detachment with retinal defect, unspecified
361.01 Recent retinal detachment, partial, with single defect
361.02 Recent retinal detachment, partial, with multiple defects
361.03 Recent retinal detachment, partial, with giant tear
361.04 Recent retinal detachment, partial, with retinal dialysis
361.05 Recent retinal detachment, total or subtotal
361.06 Old retinal detachment, partial
361.07 Old retinal detachment, total or subtotal
361.81 Traction detachment of retina

For 67028:

360.00 Purulent endophthalmitis, unspecified
360.01 Acute endophthalmitis

Applicable HCPCS Level II Codes

A4305 Disposable drug delivery system, flow rate of 50 ml or greater per hour
A4306 Disposable drug delivery system, flow rate of 5 ml or less per hour
A4550 Surgical tray

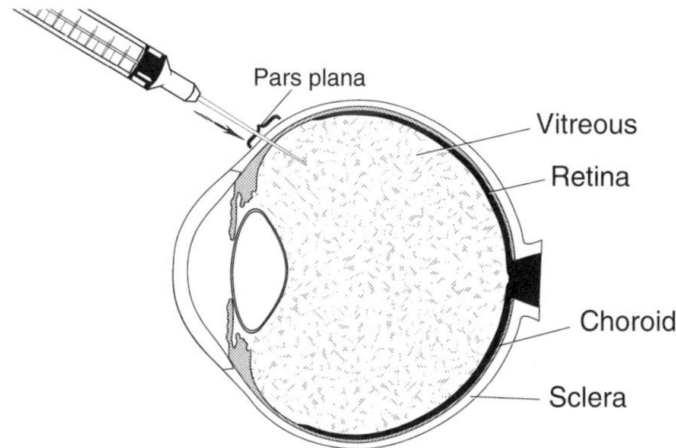

In 67025, a vitreous substitute is injected into the posterior segment; if medication is injected, report 67028 instead

CPT Description

67030 Discission of vitreous strands (without removal), pars plana approach

67031 Severing of vitreous strands, vitreous face adhesions, sheets, membranes or opacities, laser surgery (one or more stages)

Explanation

The physician makes a small incision in the conjunctiva, sclera, and choroid in the pars plana. A narrow knife is inserted to cut vitreous strands that obstruct the patient's vision (e.g., 67030) or the vitreous strands are severed by a laser (e.g., 67031). The strands generally fall away from the visual field and are not retrieved. The physician repairs the pars plana incision with a layered closure and may restore the intraocular pressure with an injection of aqueous or vitreal substitute. A cataract specialist might approach the discission through a limbal incision (at the corneal-scleral juncture), instead of through the pars plana. A topical antibiotic or pressure patch may be applied after either approach.

Comments

Code 67030 with caution: this procedure is rarely performed today because 67031 is noninvasive. For removal of corneovitreal adhesions, see 65880. This procedure is generally performed with a subconjunctival or retrobulbar injection rather than general anesthesia.

Commonly Associated ICD•9 Procedural Codes

14.79 Other operations on vitreous

Follow-up Days	Assist at Surgery
30	N

Prior Approval
N

Anesthesia Code(s)
00140

Should Not Be Billed

Not with 67030:

65270 65272 65273 65280 65285 65810 67005 67015 67025 67028 67500

Commonly Associated ICD•9 Diagnostic Codes

379.24 Other vitreous opacities
379.25 Vitreous membranes and strands
379.29 Other disorders of vitreous

Applicable HCPCS Level II Codes

A4305 Disposable drug delivery system, flow rate of 50 ml or greater per hour
A4306 Disposable drug delivery system, flow rate of 5 ml or less per hour
A4550 Surgical tray

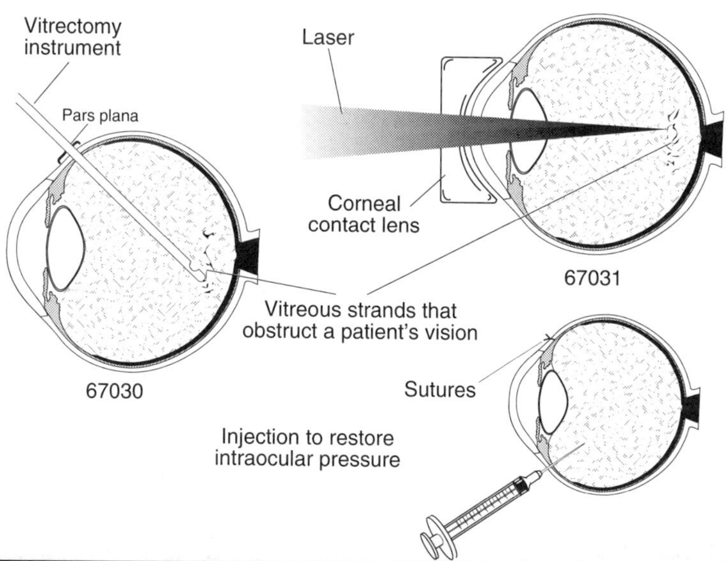

CPT Description

67036 Vitrectomy, mechanical, pars plana approach;

67038 with epiretinal membrane stripping

Explanation

The vitreous is the clear gel filling the posterior cavity of the eyeball. The physician applies a special contact lens to the cornea to can better visualize the back of the eye. Three small incisions are made in the eyeball, each about 4 mm from the juncture of the cornea and sclera. (This is the pars plana approach.) One incision is for a light cannula, one for an infusion cannula, and one for the cutting or suction instruments. The physician extracts the vitreous, using a mechanical cutting and suctioning process that may involve a special instrument like a rotoextractor or vitreous infusion suction cutter (VICS). This is often called a posterior sclerotomy in operative reports. To strip the epiretinal membrane (e.g., 67038), the physician uses a retinal cutting instrument to peel membrane or scar tissue creating tension on the retinal surface. The cannulas are extracted and the incisions repaired with layered closures. Injections may be required to reestablish intraocular pressure. A topical antibiotic or pressure patch may be applied.

Comments

For use of vitrectomy in retinal detachment surgery, see 67108. This procedure is generally performed with a retrobulbar injection rather than general anesthesia.

Commonly Associated ICD•9 Procedural Codes

14.39 Other repair of retinal tear

14.72 Other removal of vitreous

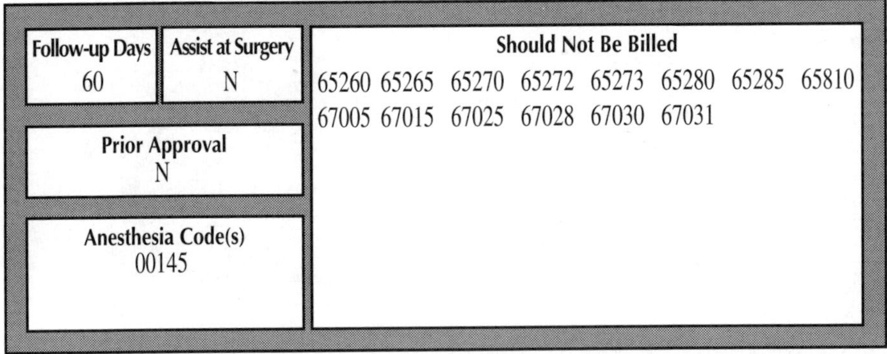

Follow-up Days	Assist at Surgery
60	N

Prior Approval
N

Anesthesia Code(s)
00145

Should Not Be Billed
65260 65265 65270 65272 65273 65280 65285 65810
67005 67015 67025 67028 67030 67031

Commonly Associated ICD•9 Diagnostic Codes

For 67036:

250.5 Diabetes with ophthalmic manifestations
360.01 Acute endophthalmitis
360.02 Panophthalmitis
360.03 Chronic endophthalmitis
360.04 Vitreous abscess
360.13 Parasitic endophthalmitis NOS
379.22 Crystalline deposits in vitreous
379.23 Vitreous hemorrhage
379.24 Other vitreous opacities
379.25 Vitreous membranes and strands
379.26 Vitreous prolapse

For 67038:

361.30 Retinal defect, unspecified
361.33 Multiple defects of retina without detachment
362.54 Macular cyst, hole, or pseudohole of retina
362.56 Macular puckering of retina
363.32 Other macular scars of retina

Applicable HCPCS Level II Codes

A4305 Disposable drug delivery system, flow rate of 50 ml or greater per hour
A4306 Disposable drug delivery system, flow rate of 5 ml or less per hour
A4550 Surgical tray

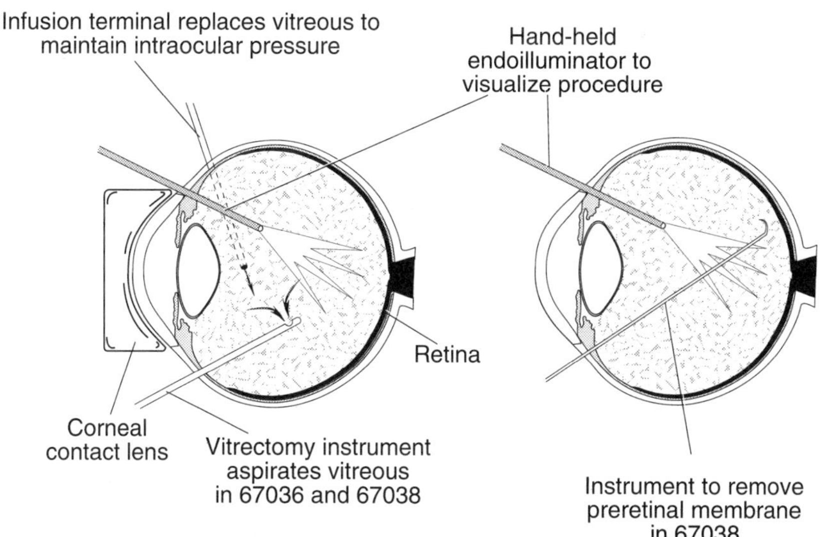

CPT Description

Vitrectomy, mechanical, pars plana approach;

67039 with focal endolaser photocoagulation

67040 endolaser panretinal photocoagulation

Explanation

The vitreous is the clear gel filling the posterior cavity of the eyeball. The physician applies a special contact lens to the cornea to can better visualize the back of the eye. Three small incisions are made in the eyeball, each about 4 mm from the juncture of the cornea and sclera. (This is the pars plana approach.) One incision is for a light cannula, one for an infusion cannula and one for the laser. The physician extracts the vitreous, using a mechanical cutting and suctioning process that may involve a special instrument like a rotoextractor or vitreous infusion suction cutter (VICS). Then, with focal endolaser photocoagulation (e.g., 67039), the physician uses a laser to treat minor retinal disorders. If the physician performs endolaser panretinal photocoagulation (e.g., 67040), a stronger laser treats larger retinal problems, like retinal detachments, diabetic retinopathy, or retinal holes. The cannulas are extracted and the incisions repaired with layered closures. Injections may be required to reestablish the intraocular pressure. A topical antibiotic or pressure patch may be applied.

Comments

For use of vitrectomy in retinal detachment surgery, see 67108. These procedures are generally performed with a retrobulbar injection rather than general anesthesia.

Commonly Associated ICD•9 Procedural Codes

14.33 Repair of retinal tear by xenon arc photocoagulation

14.34 Repair of retinal tear by laser photocoagulation

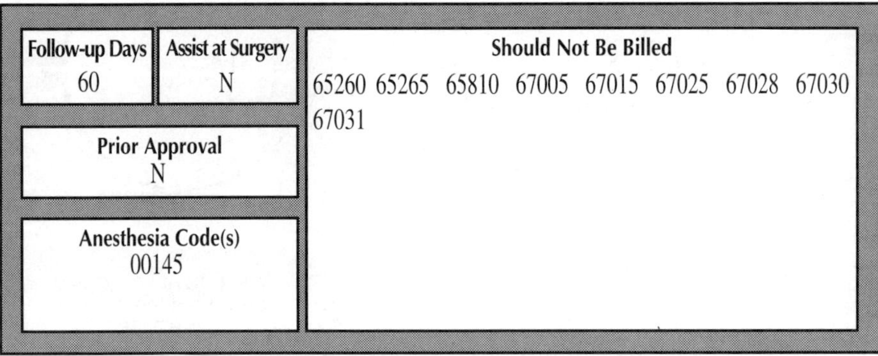

Follow-up Days	Assist at Surgery	Should Not Be Billed
60	N	65260 65265 65810 67005 67015 67025 67028 67030 67031
Prior Approval: N		
Anesthesia Code(s): 00145		

Commonly Associated ICD•9 Diagnostic Codes

361.00 Retinal detachment with retinal defect, unspecified
361.01 Recent retinal detachment, partial, with single defect
361.02 Recent retinal detachment, partial, with multiple defects
361.03 Recent retinal detachment, partial, with giant tear
361.04 Recent retinal detachment, partial, with retinal dialysis
361.05 Recent retinal detachment, total or subtotal
361.06 Old retinal detachment, partial
361.07 Old retinal detachment, total or subtotal
361.81 Traction detachment of retina
362.14 Retinal microaneurysms nos
379.24 Other vitreous opacities

For 67040:

362.01 Background diabetic retinopathy
362.02 Proliferative diabetic retinopathy

Applicable HCPCS Level II Codes

A4305 Disposable drug delivery system, flow rate of 50 ml or greater per hour
A4306 Disposable drug delivery system, flow rate of 5 ml or less per hour
A4550 Surgical tray

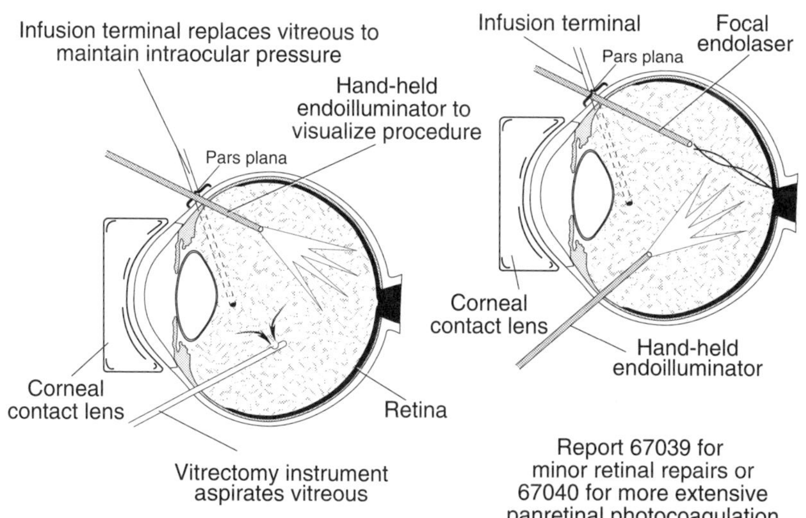

Report 67039 for minor retinal repairs or 67040 for more extensive panretinal photocoagulation

67101 CPT CODE

CPT Description

Repair of retinal detachment, one or more sessions; cryotherapy or diathermy, with or without drainage of subretinal fluid

Explanation

When the retina detaches, it separates from its nourishing blood supply and falls into the posterior cavity of the eye. Loss of vision results. The physician reattaches the retina by freezing (cryotherapy) and thus sealing the retinal tissue to the back of the eye, or by diathermy, where heat is used for the same purpose. The physician explores the sclera and stay sutures are placed under the involved rectus muscles so the eye can be rotated to expose the area to be treated. Sometimes, a rectus muscle is temporarily detached to permit adequate exposure. Cryotherapy and diathermy are performed without entering the posterior chamber; either probe is pressed against the sclera overlying the site of the retinal defect, sealing it against the choroid. If subretinal fluid must be drained, the physician makes an incision in the sclera (sclerotomy) to permit access to the middle layer of the eye's shell (the choroid), which is perforated so that fluid drains out. Any incisions are repaired with layered closures. Injections may be required to reestablish proper intraocular pressure. A topical antibiotic or pressure patch may be applied.

Comments

If diathermy, cryotherapy and/or photocoagulation are combined during a surgical session, report under the principal method. Report 67107 if this procedure is performed in conjunction with a scleral buckling. For prophylaxis of retinal detachment using cryotherapy or diathermy, see 67141. For pneumoretinopexy, see 67110. This procedure is generally performed with a retrobulbar injection rather than general anesthesia.

Commonly Associated ICD•9 Procedural Codes

14.51 Repair of retinal detachment with diathermy
14.52 Repair of retinal detachment with cryotherapy

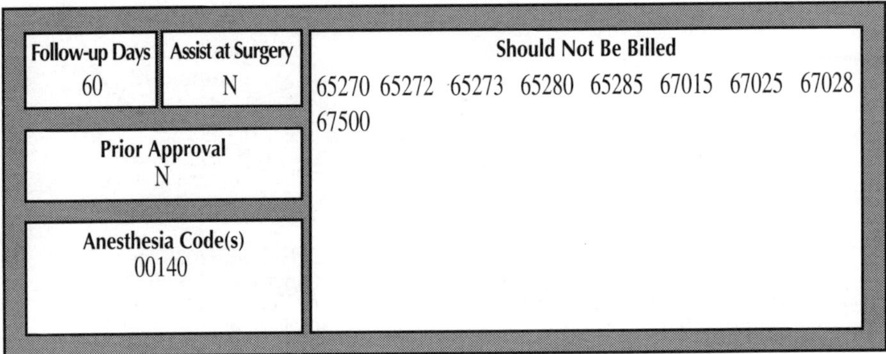

Follow-up Days	Assist at Surgery	Should Not Be Billed
60	N	65270 65272 65273 65280 65285 67015 67025 67028 67500

Prior Approval
N

Anesthesia Code(s)
00140

Commonly Associated ICD•9 Diagnostic Codes

361.00 Retinal detachment with retinal defect, unspecified
361.02 Recent retinal detachment, partial, with multiple defects
361.03 Recent retinal detachment, partial, with giant tear
361.04 Recent retinal detachment, partial, with retinal dialysis
361.05 Recent retinal detachment, total or subtotal
361.06 Old retinal detachment, partial
361.07 Old retinal detachment, total or subtotal
361.30 Retinal defect, unspecified
361.89 Other forms of retinal detachment
361.9 Unspecified retinal detachment

Applicable HCPCS Level II Codes

A4305 Disposable drug delivery system, flow rate of 50 ml or greater per hour
A4306 Disposable drug delivery system, flow rate of 5 ml or less per hour
A4550 Surgical tray

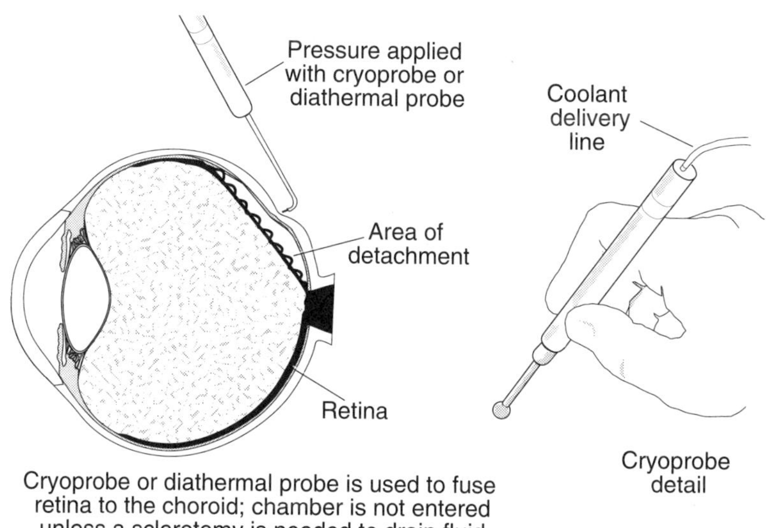

Cryoprobe or diathermal probe is used to fuse retina to the choroid; chamber is not entered unless a sclerotomy is needed to drain fluid

Detached Retina Repair

67105 CPT CODE

CPT Description

Repair of retinal detachment, one or more sessions; photocoagulation (laser or xenon arc, one or more sessions), with or without drainage of subretinal fluid

Explanation

When the retina detaches, it separates from its nourishing blood supply and falls into the posterior cavity of the eye. Loss of vision results. Using a laser light or xenon arc that goes through a dilated pupil without an incision, the physician burns spots at the site of the retinal detachment or retinal tear to seal the retina back into place against the choroid (vascular, middle layer of the eye's shell). If subretinal fluid must be drained, the physician cuts through the conjunctiva and into the sclera (sclerotomy) to access to the choroid, which is perforated so that fluid drains out. Any incisions are repaired with layered closures. Injections may be required to reestablish the intraocular pressure. A topical antibiotic or pressure patch may be applied.

Comments

If laser therapy is combined with cryotherapy or diathermy, the dominant procedure should be billed. This procedure is generally performed with a topical anesthetic rather than general anesthesia.

Commonly Associated ICD•9 Procedural Codes

14.53 Repair of retinal detachment with xenon arc photocoagulation

14.54 Repair of retinal detachment with laser photocoagulation

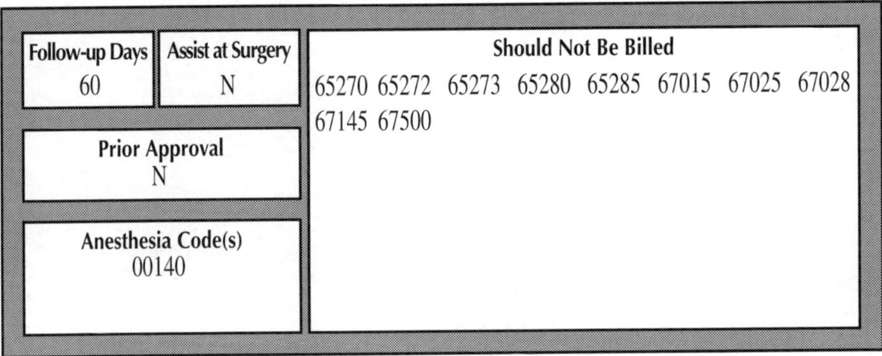

Follow-up Days	Assist at Surgery
60	N

Prior Approval
N

Anesthesia Code(s)
00140

Should Not Be Billed
65270 65272 65273 65280 65285 67015 67025 67028 67145 67500

Commonly Associated ICD•9 Diagnostic Codes

361.00 Retinal detachment with retinal defect, unspecified
361.01 Recent retinal detachment, partial, with single defect
361.02 Recent retinal detachment, partial, with multiple defects
361.03 Recent retinal detachment, partial, with giant tear
361.04 Recent retinal detachment, partial, with retinal dialysis
361.05 Recent retinal detachment, total or subtotal
361.06 Old retinal detachment, partial
361.07 Old retinal detachment, total or subtotal
361.2 Serous retinal detachment
361.89 Other forms of retinal detachment
361.9 Unspecified retinal detachment

Applicable HCPCS Level II Codes

A4305 Disposable drug delivery system, flow rate of 50 ml or greater per hour
A4306 Disposable drug delivery system, flow rate of 5 ml or less per hour
A4550 Surgical tray

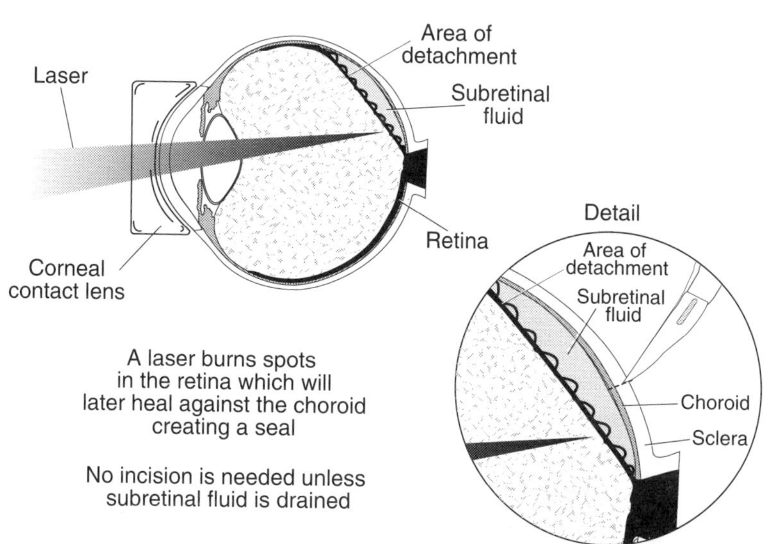

67107 CPT CODE

CPT Description

Repair of retinal detachment, one or more sessions; scleral buckling (such as lamellar excision, imbrication or encircling procedure), with or without implant, may include procedures 67101, 67105

Explanation

The physician explores the sclera to locate the site overlying a retinal detachment. Stay sutures are placed under involves rectus muscles so the eye may be exposed to area that will be treated. The physician treats the retinal tear externally, by placing a cold or hot probe over the scleral and depressing it. The burn seals the choroid to the retina at the site of the tear. The physician cuts a groove in the sclera and mattress sutures are places across this incision. Any subretinal fluid is drained. A Silastic band is laid in the scleral bed and sutured in place. Sometimes, a silicone patch is placed under the band. Additional cryotherapy or diathermy may be accomplished at this time. When the tear has been adequately repaired and supported, the rectus muscle sutures are removed.

Comments

See 67250 for scleral reinforcement. This procedure is generally performed with a subconjunctival o injection rather than general anesthesia.

Commonly Associated ICD•9 Procedural Codes

14.41 Scleral buckling with implant

14.49 Other scleral buckling

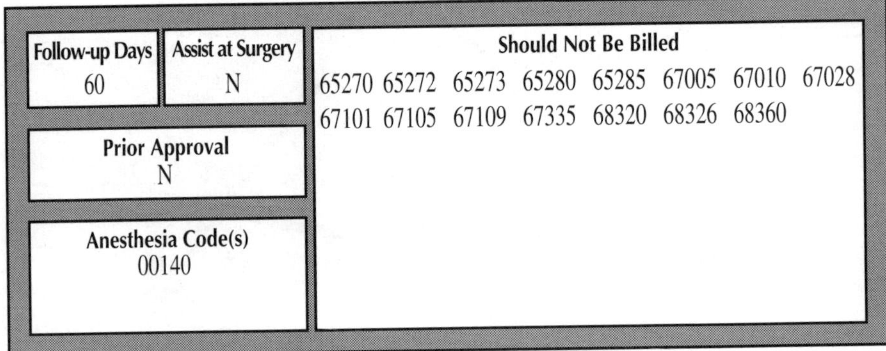

Follow-up Days	Assist at Surgery	Prior Approval	Anesthesia Code(s)
60	N	N	00140

Should Not Be Billed

65270 65272 65273 65280 65285 67005 67010 67028 67101 67105 67109 67335 68320 68326 68360

Commonly Associated ICD•9 Diagnostic Codes

361.00 Retinal detachment with retinal defect, unspecified
361.01 Recent retinal detachment, partial, with single defect
361.02 Recent retinal detachment, partial, with multiple defects
361.03 Recent retinal detachment, partial, with giant tear
361.04 Recent retinal detachment, partial, with retinal dialysis
361.05 Recent retinal detachment, total or subtotal
361.06 Old retinal detachment, partial
361.07 Old retinal detachment, total or subtotal
361.89 Other forms of retinal detachment
361.9 Unspecified retinal detachment

Applicable HCPCS Level II Codes

A4305 Disposable drug delivery system, flow rate of 50 ml or greater per hour
A4306 Disposable drug delivery system, flow rate of 5 ml or less per hour
A4550 Surgical tray

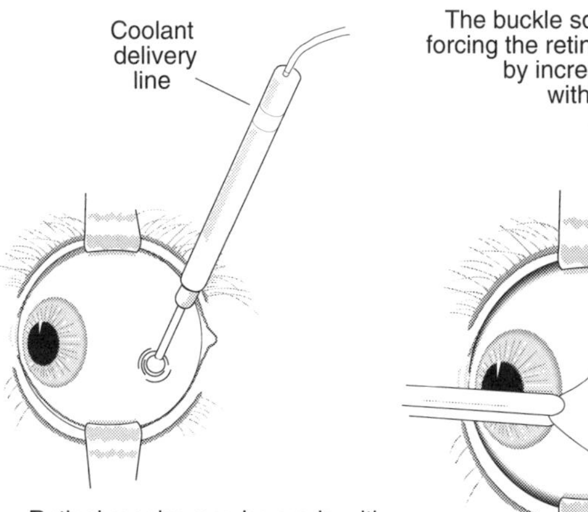

67108 CPT CODE

CPT Description

Repair of retinal detachment, one or more sessions; with vitrectomy, any method, with or without air or gas tamponade, with or without focal endolaser photocoagulation, may include procedures 67101-67107 and/or removal of lens by same technique

Explanation

When the retina detaches, it separates from its nourishing blood supply and falls into the posterior cavity of the eye. Loss of vision results. The physician reattaches the retina by freezing (cryotherapy) and thus sealing the retinal tissue to the back of the eye, by diathermy, where heat is used for the same purpose, or by laser. Cryotherapy and diathermy are performed without entering the posterior chamber; either probe is pressed against the sclera overlying the site of the retinal defect, sealing it against the choroid. If a laser is used, the light goes through a dilated pupil without an incision to burn spots at the site of the retinal detachment or retinal tear to seal the retina back into place against the choroid (vascular, middle layer of the eye's shell). A scleral buckle may be placed. The physician removes any vitreous opacity or vitreous traction. The lens may also be removed if it interferes with the physician's view of the retina or if the lens is in the way of the removal of scar tissue. Any incisions may be repaired with sutures. Antibiotic ointment and a pressure patch may be applied.

Comments

This procedure is generally performed with a subconjunctival injection rather than general anesthesia.

Commonly Associated ICD•9 Procedural Codes

14.51 Repair of retinal detachment with diathermy
14.52 Repair of retinal detachment with cryotherapy

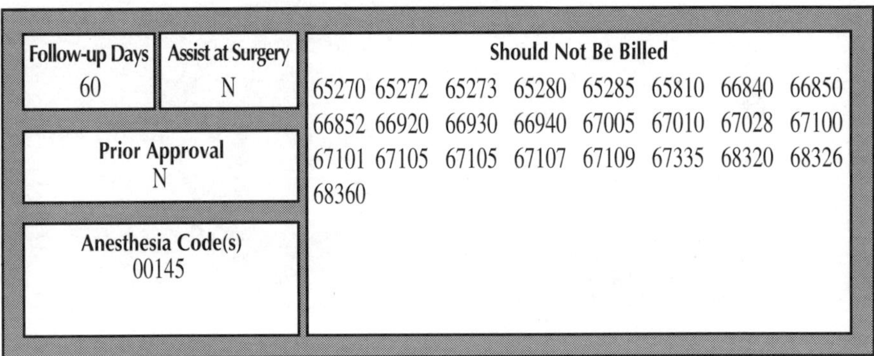

Follow-up Days	Assist at Surgery
60	N

Prior Approval
N

Anesthesia Code(s)
00145

Should Not Be Billed

65270 65272 65273 65280 65285 65810 66840 66850
66852 66920 66930 66940 67005 67010 67028 67100
67101 67105 67105 67107 67109 67335 68320 68326
68360

Commonly Associated ICD•9 Diagnostic Codes

361.00 Retinal detachment with retinal defect, unspecified
361.01 Recent retinal detachment, partial, with single defect
361.02 Recent retinal detachment, partial, with multiple defects
361.03 Recent retinal detachment, partial, with giant tear
361.04 Recent retinal detachment, partial, with retinal dialysis
361.05 Recent retinal detachment, total or subtotal
361.06 Old retinal detachment, partial
361.07 Old retinal detachment, total or subtotal
361.89 Other forms of retinal detachment
361.9 Unspecified retinal detachment

Applicable HCPCS Level II Codes

å4305 Disposable drug delivery system, flow rate of 50 ml or greater per hour
A4306 Disposable drug delivery system, flow rate of 5 ml or less per hour
A4550 Surgical tray

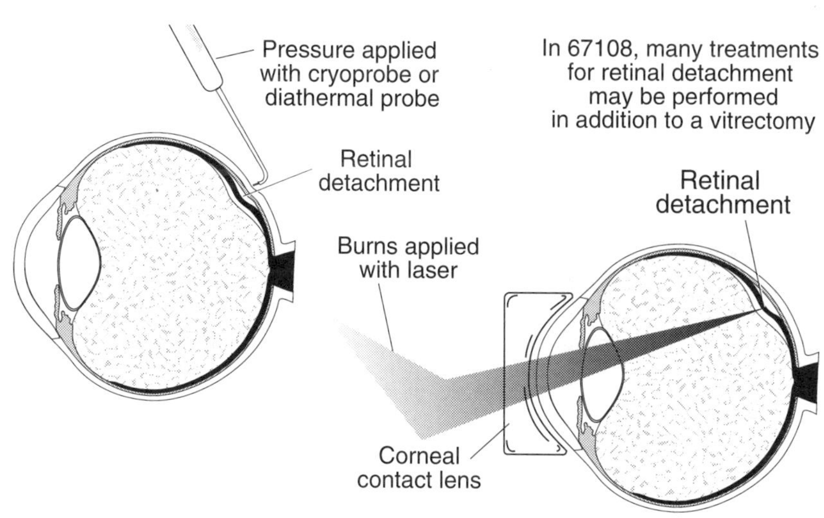

Detached Retina Repair

67110 CPT CODE

CPT Description

Repair of retinal detachment, one or more sessions; by injection of air or other gas (eg, pneumoretinopexy)

Explanation

When the retina detaches, it separates from its nourishing blood supply and falls into the posterior cavity of the eye. Loss of vision results. The physician uses a needle to inject expandable gas into the eye to flatten the retinal tear, then applies laser or cryotherapy to seal the retinal tear. The physician explores the sclera to locate the site overlying a retinal detachment. Stay sutures are placed under involves rectus muscles so the eye may be exposed to area that will be treated. Air or other gas is injected through the sclera into the posterior segment of the eye to flatten the retinal detachment against the choroid (The patient is instructed to maintain a posture that will position the bubble against the detachment.) The physician treats the retinal tear externally, by placing a cold (cryotherapy) or hot (diathermy) probe over the sclera and depressing it. The burn seals the choroid to the retina at the site of the tear. This procedure is often called pneumatic retinopexy.

Comments

This procedure is reported only once even if repeated during the global period. This procedure is generally performed with a subconjunctival or retrobulbar injection rather than general anesthesia.

Commonly Associated ICD•9 Procedural Codes

14.59 Other repair of retinal detachment

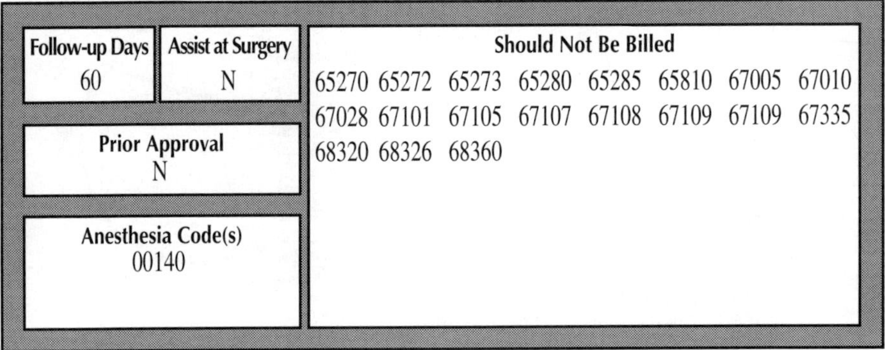

Follow-up Days	Assist at Surgery
60	N

Prior Approval
N

Anesthesia Code(s)
00140

Should Not Be Billed

65270 65272 65273 65280 65285 65810 67005 67010
67028 67101 67105 67107 67108 67109 67109 67335
68320 68326 68360

Commonly Associated ICD•9 Diagnostic Codes

361.00 Retinal detachment with retinal defect, unspecified
361.01 Recent retinal detachment, partial, with single defect
361.02 Recent retinal detachment, partial, with multiple defects
361.03 Recent retinal detachment, partial, with giant tear
361.04 Recent retinal detachment, partial, with retinal dialysis
361.05 Recent retinal detachment, total or subtotal
361.06 Old retinal detachment, partial
361.07 Old retinal detachment, total or subtotal
361.89 Other forms of retinal detachment
361.9 Unspecified retinal detachment

Applicable HCPCS Level II Codes

A4305 Disposable drug delivery system, flow rate of 50 ml or greater per hour
A4306 Disposable drug delivery system, flow rate of 5 ml or less per hour
A4550 Surgical tray

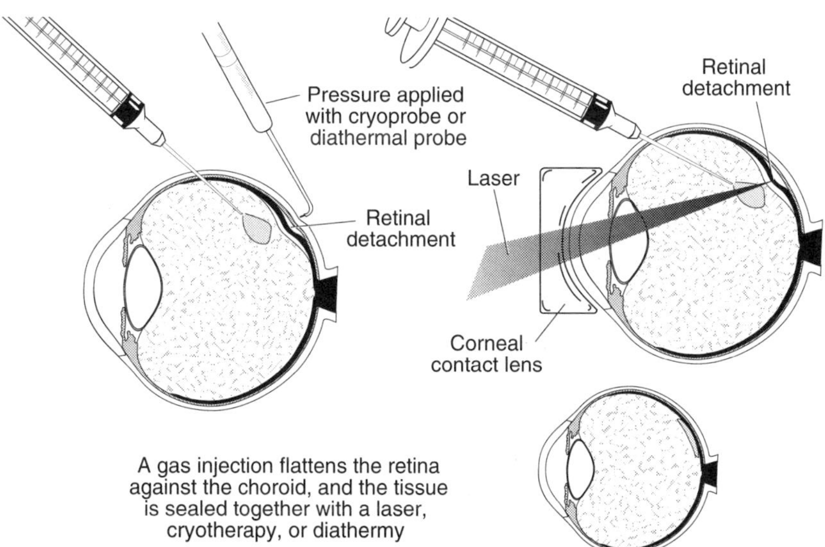

A gas injection flattens the retina against the choroid, and the tissue is sealed together with a laser, cryotherapy, or diathermy

Detached Retina Repair

67115 CPT CODE

CPT Description

Release of encircling material (posterior segment)

Explanation

The physician inserts an ocular speculum. To release tension of a previously placed scleral buckle, the physician makes an incision in the conjunctiva and sclera, adjusts the buckle and repairs the surgical wound with sutures.

Comments

To report the removal of other implanted materials in the posterior segment, use 67120. This procedure is generally performed with a subconjunctival injection rather than general anesthesia.

Commonly Associated ICD•9 Procedural Codes

14.6 Removal of surgically implanted material from posterior segment of eye

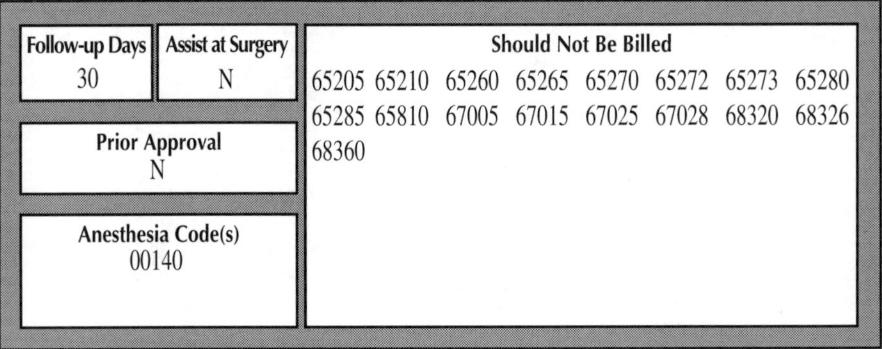

Follow-up Days	Assist at Surgery
30	N

Prior Approval
N

Anesthesia Code(s)
00140

Should Not Be Billed
65205 65210 65260 65265 65270 65272 65273 65280
65285 65810 67005 67015 67025 67028 68320 68326
68360

Commonly Associated ICD•9 Diagnostic Codes

365.89 Other specified glaucoma
368.2 Diplopia
378.6 Mechanical strabismus
V45.6 Postsurgical states following surgery of eye and adnexa

Applicable HCPCS Level II Codes

A4305 Disposable drug delivery system, flow rate of 50 ml or greater per hour
A4306 Disposable drug delivery system, flow rate of 5 ml or less per hour
A4550 Surgical tray

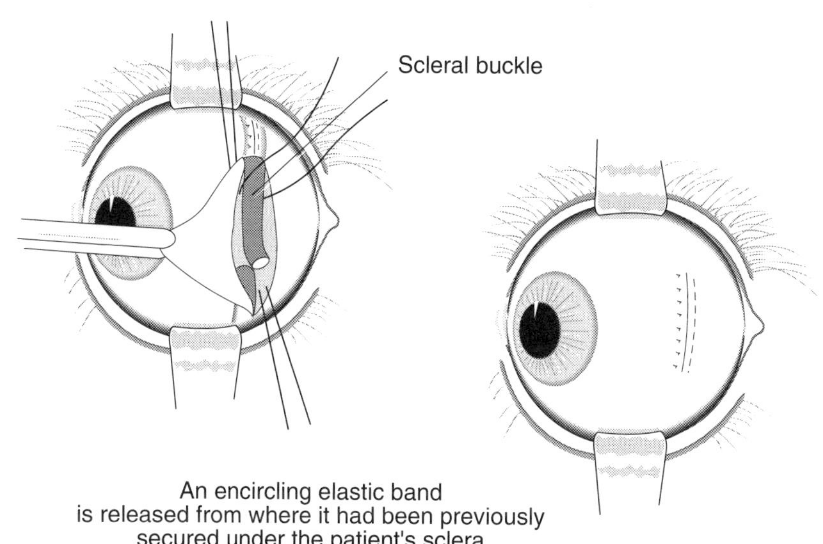

An encircling elastic band is released from where it had been previously secured under the patient's sclera

Scleral Buckle Release

67120 CPT CODE

CPT Description

Removal of implanted material, posterior segment; extraocular

Explanation

The physician inserts an ocular speculum. The physician removes a previously implanted extraocular tube, reservoir, buckle, or other prosthetic device from the eye. The physician may close the incision with sutures and may restore the intraocular pressure with an injection of water or saline. A topical antibiotic or pressure patch may be applied.

Comments

Use 65920 if haptic of anterior intraocular lens is removed. This procedure is generally performed with a subconjunctival injection rather than general anesthesia.

Commonly Associated ICD•9 Procedural Codes

14.6 Removal of surgically implanted material from posterior segment of eye

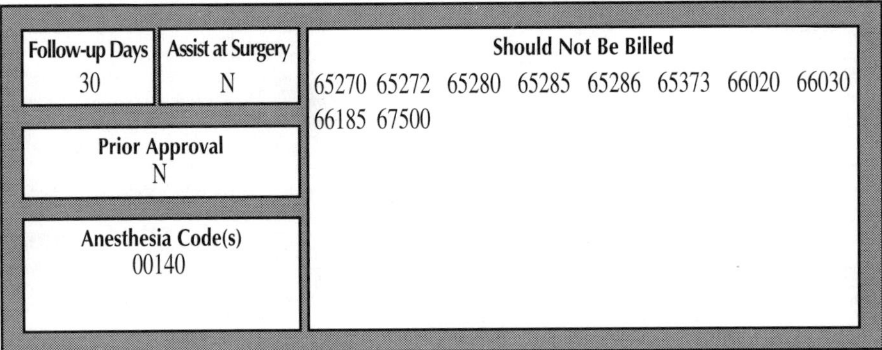

Follow-up Days	Assist at Surgery	Should Not Be Billed
30	N	65270 65272 65280 65285 65286 65373 66020 66030 66185 67500
Prior Approval: N		
Anesthesia Code(s): 00140		

Commonly Associated ICD•9 Diagnostic Codes

361.00 Retinal detachment with retinal defect, unspecified
361.01 Recent retinal detachment, partial, with single defect
361.02 Recent retinal detachment, partial, with multiple defects
361.03 Recent retinal detachment, partial, with giant tear
361.04 Recent retinal detachment, partial, with retinal dialysis
361.05 Recent retinal detachment, total or subtotal
361.06 Old retinal detachment, partial
361.07 Old retinal detachment, total or subtotal
361.89 Other forms of retinal detachment
368.2 Diplopia
378.60 Mechanical strabismus
V45.6 Postsurgical states following surgery of eye and adnexa

Applicable HCPCS Level II Codes

A4305 Disposable drug delivery system, flow rate of 50 ml or greater per hour
A4306 Disposable drug delivery system, flow rate of 5 ml or less per hour
A4550 Surgical tray

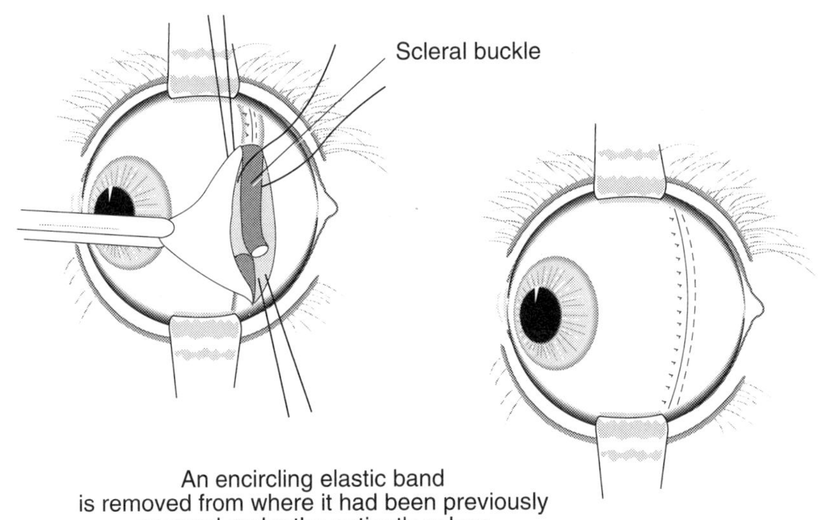

An encircling elastic band is removed from where it had been previously secured under the patient's sclera

67121 CPT CODE

CPT Description

Removal of implanted material, posterior segment; intraocular

Explanation

An incision is made in the pars plana near the site of an intraocular lens that has fallen into the posterior segment of the eye. The physician then removes the extracapsular IOL from the eye. The physician closes the incision with sutures and may restore the intraocular pressure with an injection of vitreous substitute. A topical antibiotic or pressure patch may be applied.

Comments

If a lens is removed from the anterior sefment, report 65920. This procedure may be performed with a retrobulbar injection rather than general anesthesia.

Commonly Associated ICD•9 Procedural Codes

13.8 Removal of implanted lens

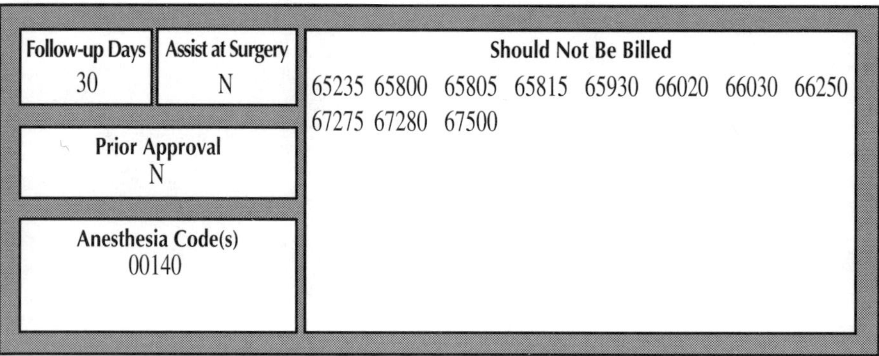

Follow-up Days	Assist at Surgery	Should Not Be Billed
30	N	65235 65800 65805 65815 65930 66020 66030 66250 67275 67280 67500

Prior Approval
N

Anesthesia Code(s)
00140

Commonly Associated ICD•9 Diagnostic Codes

379.32 Subluxation of lens
379.34 Posterior dislocation of lens
379.39 Other disorders of lens
V45.6 Postsurgical states following surgery of eye and adnexa

Applicable HCPCS Level II Codes

A4305 Disposable drug delivery system, flow rate of 50 ml or greater per hour
A4306 Disposable drug delivery system, flow rate of 5 ml or less per hour
A4550 Surgical tray

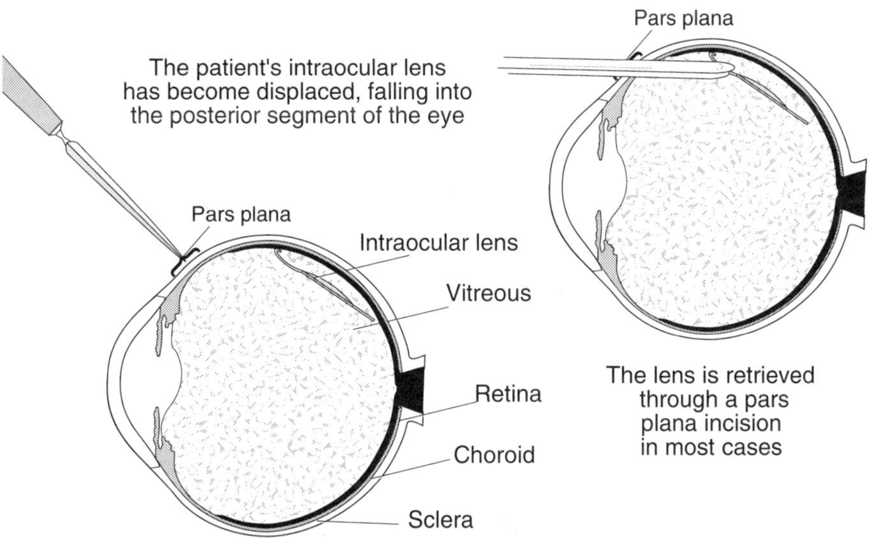

IOL REMOVAL

67141 CPT CODE

CPT Description

Prophylaxis of retinal detachment (eg, retinal break, lattice degeneration) without drainage, one or more sessions; cryotherapy, diathermy

Explanation

When the retina detaches, it separates from its nourishing blood supply and falls into the posterior cavity of the eye. Loss of vision results. The physician secures a degenerating retina by freezing (cryotherapy) and thus sealing the retinal tissue to the back of the eye, or by diathermy, where heat is used for the same purpose. The physician explores the sclera and stay sutures are placed under the involved rectus muscles so the eye can be rotated to expose the area to be treated. Sometimes, a rectus muscle is temporarily detached to permit adequate exposure. Cryotherapy and diathermy are performed without entering the posterior chamber; either probe is pressed against the sclera overlying the site of the retinal defect, sealing it against the choroid.

Comments

Multiple sessions of this service are reported once during the global period. This procedure is generally performed with a subconjunctival inject… or topical anesthetic rather than general anesthesia.

Commonly Associated ICD•9 Procedural Codes

14.31 Repair of retinal tear by diathermy
14.32 Repair of retinal tear by cryotherapy

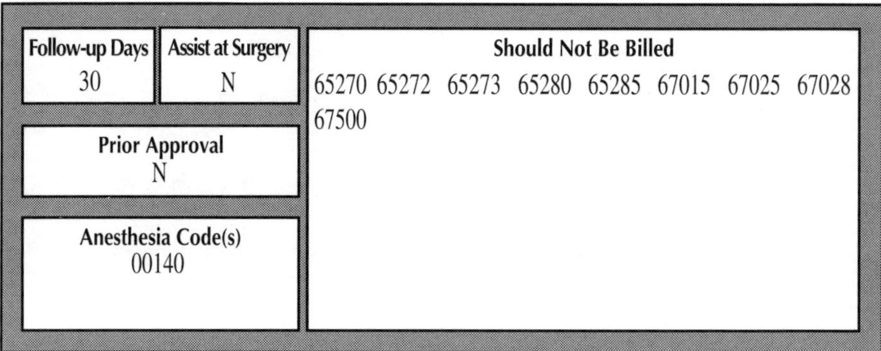

Follow-up Days	Assist at Surgery	Should Not Be Billed
30	N	65270 65272 65273 65280 65285 67015 67025 67028 67500

Prior Approval
N

Anesthesia Code(s)
00140

Commonly Associated ICD•9 Diagnostic Codes

361.00 Retinal detachment with retinal defect, unspecified
361.01 Recent retinal detachment, partial, with single defect
361.02 Recent retinal detachment, partial, with multiple defects
361.03 Recent retinal detachment, partial, with giant tear
361.04 Recent retinal detachment, partial, with retinal dialysis
361.05 Recent retinal detachment, total or subtotal
361.06 Old retinal detachment, partial
361.07 Old retinal detachment, total or subtotal
362.63 Lattice degeneration of retina

Applicable HCPCS Level II Codes

A4305 Disposable drug delivery system, flow rate of 50 ml or greater per hour
A4306 Disposable drug delivery system, flow rate of 5 ml or less per hour
A4550 Surgical tray

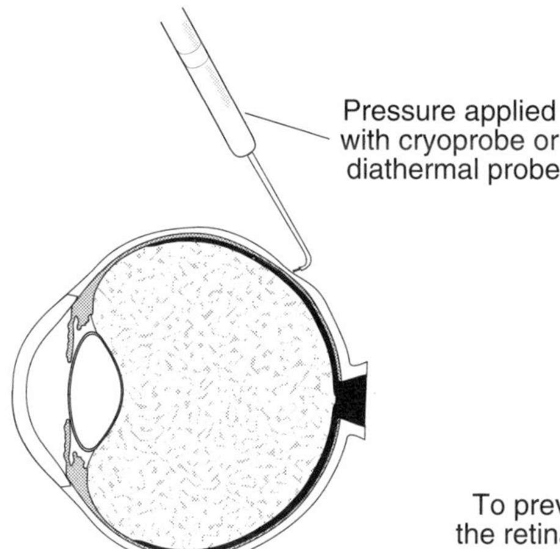

To prevent retinal detachment, the retina is sealed to the choroid tissue underlying it

67145 CPT CODE

CPT Description

Prophylaxis of retinal detachment (eg, retinal break, lattice degeneration) without drainage, one or more sessions; photocoagulation (laser or xenon arc)

Explanation

Using a laser light or xenon arc that goes through a dilated pupil without an incision, the physician burns spots at the site of the retinal weakness to seal the retina into place against the choroid (vascular, middle layer of the eye's shell). No incision is made. Multiple sessions may be required.

Comments

Multiple sessions of this service are reported once during the global period. This procedure is generally performed with a topical anesthetic rather than general anesthesia.

Commonly Associated ICD•9 Procedural Codes

14.33 Repair of retinal tear by xenon arc photocoagulation

14.34 Repair of retinal tear by laser photocoagulation

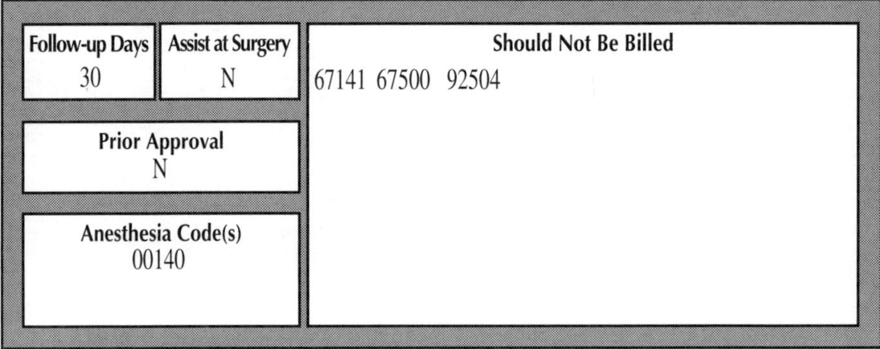

Follow-up Days	Assist at Surgery	Should Not Be Billed
30	N	67141 67500 92504

Prior Approval
N

Anesthesia Code(s)
00140

Commonly Associated ICD•9 Diagnostic Codes

361.00 Retinal detachment with retinal defect, unspecified
361.01 Recent retinal detachment, partial, with single defect
361.01 Recent retinal detachment, partial, with single defect
361.02 Recent retinal detachment, partial, with multiple defects
361.03 Recent retinal detachment, partial, with giant tear
361.04 Recent retinal detachment, partial, with retinal dialysis
361.05 Recent retinal detachment, total or subtotal
361.06 Old retinal detachment, partial
361.07 Old retinal detachment, total or subtotal
362.63 Lattice degeneration of retina

Applicable HCPCS Level II Codes

A4305 Disposable drug delivery system, flow rate of 50 ml or greater per hour
A4306 Disposable drug delivery system, flow rate of 5 ml or less per hour
A4550 Surgical tray

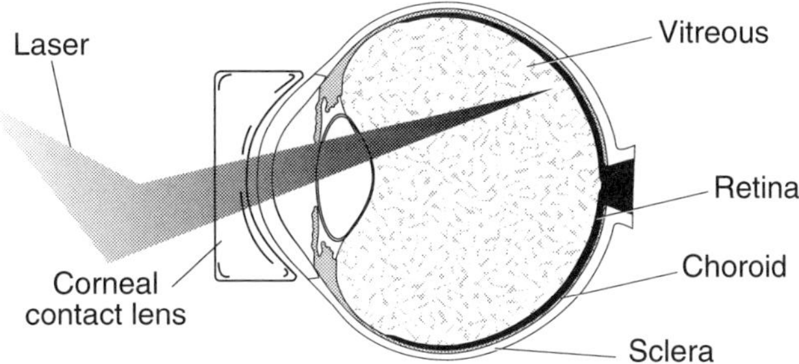

No incision is made in this procedure

Heat from the laser seals the retina to the choroid behind it, preventing a retinal detachment

67208 CPT CODE

CPT Description

Destruction of localized lesion of retina (eg, maculopathy, choroidopathy, small tumors), one or more sessions; cryotherapy, diathermy

Explanation

The physician destroys a lesion of the retina by freezing (cryotherapy) , or by heat (diathermy). The physician explores the sclera and stay sutures are placed under the involves rectus muscles so the eye can be rotated to expose the area to be treated. Sometimes, a rectus muscle is temporarily detached to permit adequate exposure. Cryotherapy and diathermy are performed without entering the posterior chamber; either probe is pressed against the sclera overlying the site of the retinal lesion until it is destroyed or until the session is completed. Any muscle incision is repaired and any stay sutures removed. A topical antibiotic or pressure patch may be applied.

Comments

Code with caution: this procedure has largely been replaced by laser surgery. Multiple sessions of this service are reported once during the global period. No tissue is removed in this procedure. For photocoagulation, see 67210. This procedure is generally performed with a subconjunctival or retrobulbar injection rather than general anesthesia.

Commonly Associated ICD•9 Procedural Codes

14.21 Destruction of chorioretinal lesion by diathermy

14.22 Destruction of chorioretinal lesion by cryotherapy

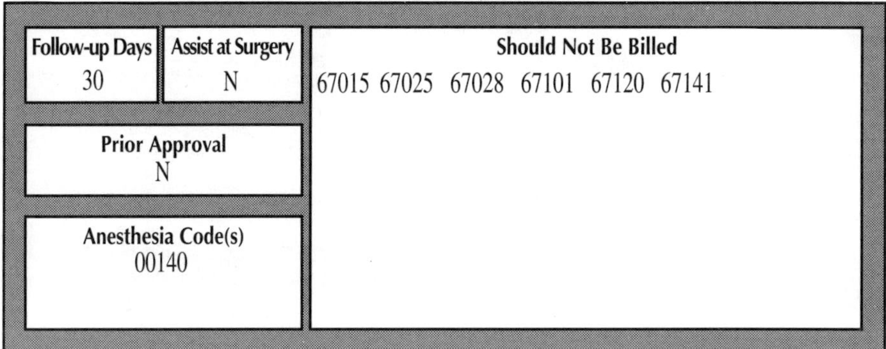

Follow-up Days	Assist at Surgery	Should Not Be Billed
30	N	67015 67025 67028 67101 67120 67141

Prior Approval
N

Anesthesia Code(s)
00140

Commonly Associated ICD•9 Diagnostic Codes

190.5 Malignant neoplasm of retina
190.6 Malignant neoplasm of choroid
224.5 Benign neoplasm of retina
224.6 Benign neoplasm of choroid

Applicable HCPCS Level II Codes

A4305 Disposable drug delivery system, flow rate of 50 ml or greater per hour
A4306 Disposable drug delivery system, flow rate of 5 ml or less per hour
A4550 Surgical tray

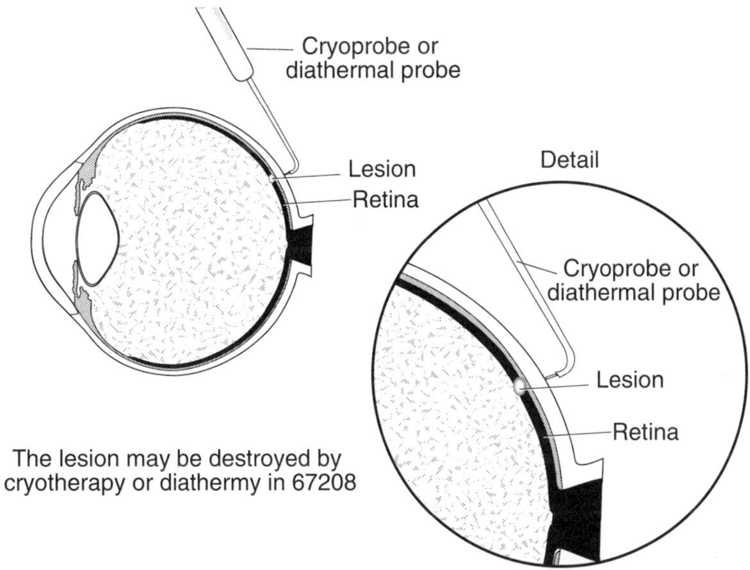

The lesion may be destroyed by cryotherapy or diathermy in 67208

67210 CPT CODE

CPT Description

Destruction of localized lesion of retina (eg, maculopathy, choroidopathy, small tumors), one or more sessions; photocoagulation (laser or xenon arc)

Explanation

The physician destroys a lesion of the retina using a laser or xenon arc. After the patient's eye has been dilated, the physician places a special contact on the eye of the patient. Photocoagulation is performed without entering the posterior chamber; the destructive light beam is guided through the contact and to the retinal lesion, which is destroyed in one session or in a series of sessions. A topical antibiotic or pressure patch may be applied.

Comments

Multiple sessions of this service are reported once during the global period. For cryotherapy or diathermy, see 67208. This procedure is generally performed with a topical anesthetic rather than general anesthesia.

Commonly Associated ICD•9 Procedural Codes

14.23 Destruction of chorioretinal lesion by xenon arc photocoagulation

14.24 Destruction of chorioretinal lesion by laser photocoagulation

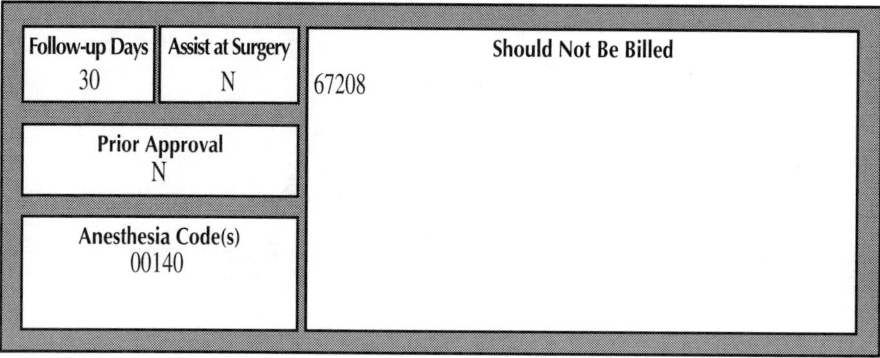

Follow-up Days	Assist at Surgery	Should Not Be Billed
30	N	67208

Prior Approval
N

Anesthesia Code(s)
00140

Commonly Associated ICD•9 Diagnostic Codes

190.5 Malignant neoplasm of retina
224.5 Benign neoplasm of retina
224.6 Benign neoplasm of choroid
362.01 Background diabetic retinopathy
362.02 Proliferative diabetic retinopathy
362.12 Exudative retinopathy
362.3 Retinal vascular occlusion
362.35 Central retinal vein occlusion
362.42 Serous detachment of retinal pigment epithelium
362.43 Hemorrhagic detachment of retinal pigment epithelium
362.52 Exudative senile macular degeneration of retina
362.54 Macular cyst, hole, or pseudohole of retina
362.82 Retinal exudates and deposits
363.40 Choroidal degeneration, unspecified

Applicable HCPCS Level II Codes

A4305 Disposable drug delivery system, flow rate of 50 ml or greater per hour
A4306 Disposable drug delivery system, flow rate of 5 ml or less per hour
A4550 Surgical tray

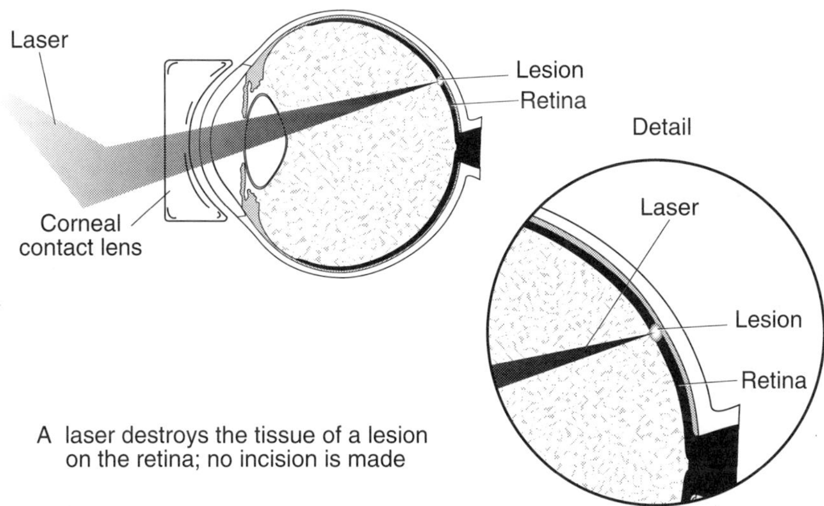

A laser destroys the tissue of a lesion on the retina; no incision is made

67218 CPT CODE

CPT Description

Destruction of localized lesion of retina (eg, maculopathy, choroidopathy, small tumors), one or more sessions; radiation by implantation of source (includes removal of source)

Explanation

The physician treats a malignancy by exposing it to a radioactive implant. The plaque-like implant is secured with sutures to the sclera overlying the site of a malignancy. At a future time, the physician recovers the implant. The incision is repaired. An antibiotic ointment and pressure patch may be applied.

Comments

The retrieval of the implant is included as part of this procedure and should not be separately reported. This procedure is generally performed with a retrobulbar injection rather than general anesthesia.

Commonly Associated ICD•9 Procedural Codes

14.27 Destruction of chorioretinal lesion by implantation of radiation source

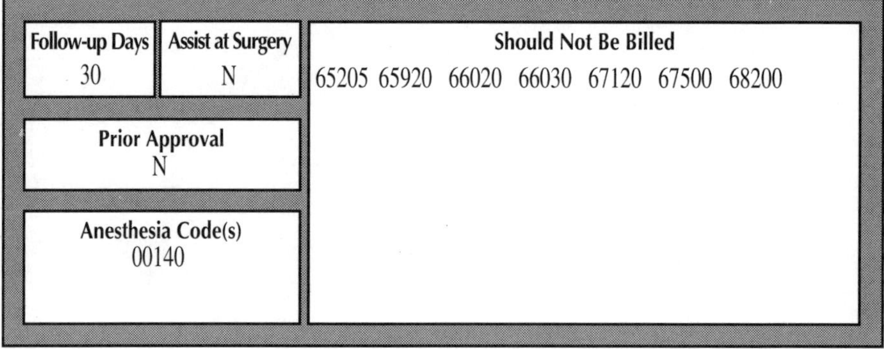

Follow-up Days	Assist at Surgery
30	N

Prior Approval
N

Anesthesia Code(s)
00140

Should Not Be Billed
65205 65920 66020 66030 67120 67500 68200

Commonly Associated ICD•9 Diagnostic Codes

190.5 Malignant neoplasm of retina
190.6 Malignant neoplasm of choroid
224.5 Benign neoplasm of retina
224.6 Benign neoplasm of choroid

Applicable HCPCS Level II Codes

A4305 Disposable drug delivery system, flow rate of 50 ml or greater per hour
A4306 Disposable drug delivery system, flow rate of 5 ml or less per hour
A4550 Surgical tray

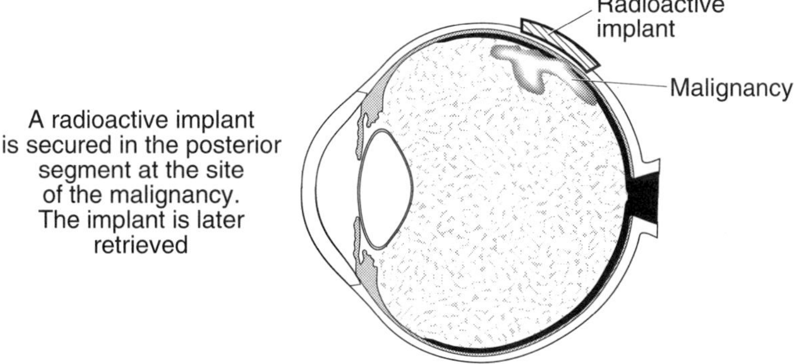

67218 describes an implantation treatment for malignancy

CPT Description

67227 Destruction of extensive or progressive retinopathy (eg, diabetic retinopathy), one or more sessions; cryotherapy, diathermy

67228 photocoagulation (laser or xenon arc)

Explanation

The physician destroys small vessels that are leaking blood on the retina by freezing (cryotherapy) , or by heat (diathermy) (e.g., 67227), or by laser (e.g., 67228). Cryotherapy and diathermy may be performed without entering the posterior chamber; either probe is pressed against the sclera overlying the site of the retinopathy until it is destroyed. With a laser light or xenon arc aimed through a dilated pupil without an incision, the physician may burn spots at the site of diabetic retinopathy to seal vessels that have been leaking into the retina. At least 500 Xenon arc burns o or 2000 burns from an argon laser are applied. This procedure is often referred to as "scattered destruction." Multiple sessions may be required.

Comments

Treatment of one eye at a time is recommended in bilateral disease. Multiple sessions of this service are reported once during the global period. This procedure is generally performed with a topical anesthetic or subconjunctival injection rather than general anesthesia.

Commonly Associated ICD•9 Procedural Codes

14.23 Destruction of chorioretinal lesion by xenon arc photocoagulation

14.24 Destruction of chorioretinal lesion by laser photocoagulation

14.9 Other operations on retina, choroid, and posterior chamber

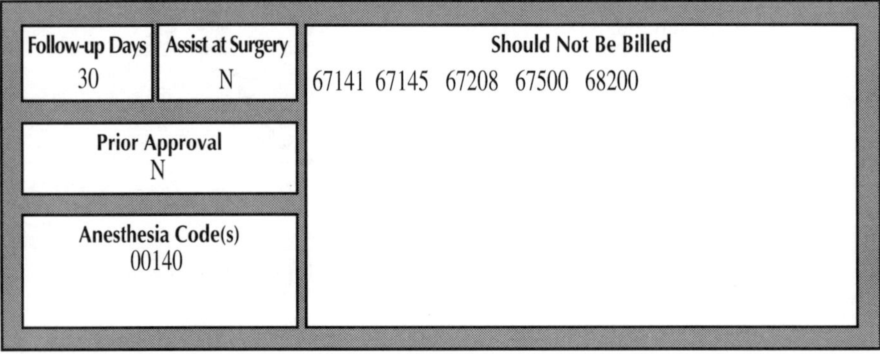

Follow-up Days	Assist at Surgery	Should Not Be Billed
30	N	67141 67145 67208 67500 68200

Prior Approval
N

Anesthesia Code(s)
00140

Commonly Associated ICD•9 Diagnostic Codes

250.50 Type II diabetes mellitus with ophthalmic manifestations
250.51 Type I diabetes mellitus with ophthalmic manifestations
362.01 Background diabetic retinopathy
362.02 Proliferative diabetic retinopathy
362.21 Retrolental fibroplasia
362.29 Other nondiabetic proliferative retinopathy

Applicable HCPCS Level II Codes

A4305 Disposable drug delivery system, flow rate of 50 ml or greater per hour
A4306 Disposable drug delivery system, flow rate of 5 ml or less per hour
A4550 Surgical tray

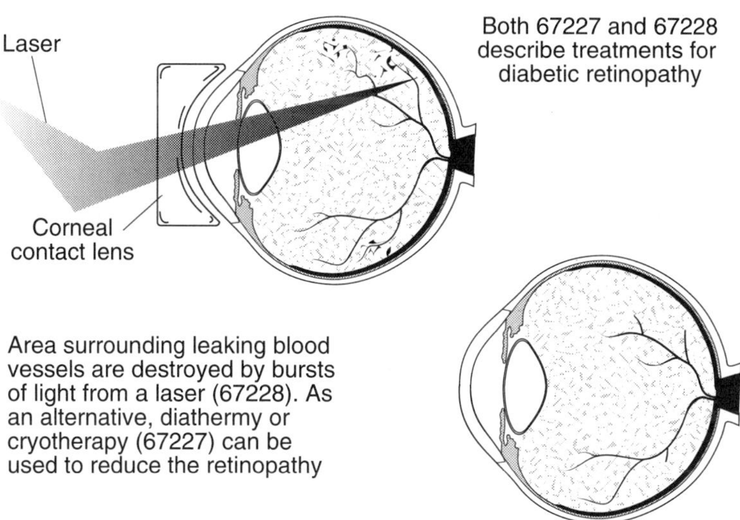

CPT Description

67250 Scleral reinforcement (separate procedure); without graft

67255 with graft

Explanation

To repair a thin, weakened sclera, the physician places an ocular speculum in the patient's eye, and makes an incision in the conjunctiva and sclera over the site of the defect. The sclera may be cinched and overlapped for reinforcement (e.g., for 67250) or a patch of donor sclera may be sutured over the weakened area (e.g., 67255). A piece of stretched sclera may also be removed. The physician uses sutures or tissue glue in the layered repair. Antibiotic ointment and a patch may be applied.

Comments

For repair of a protrusion of the contents of the eyeball at a point where the sclera has become too thin (scleral staphyloma), see 66220, 66225. For repair of a protrusion of the contents of the eyeball at a point where the sclera has become too thin (scleral staphyloma), see 66220, 66225. As a separate procedure, this procedure is usually an intrinsic part of a more complex service, and therefore is not reportable. However, when performed separately and for a specific purpose, it can be reported separately. This procedure is generally performed with a subconjunctival injection rather than general anesthesia.

Commonly Associated ICD•9 Procedural Codes

12.87 Scleral reinforcement with graft

12.88 Other scleral reinforcement

Follow-up Days	Assist at Surgery
30	N

Prior Approval
N

Anesthesia Code(s)
00140

Should Not Be Billed

65270	65272	65273	65280	65285	65286	66130	66220
66225	66250	67015	67025	67028	68200	68360	68362

Commonly Associated ICD•9 Diagnostic Codes

871.0 Ocular laceration without prolapse of intraocular tissue
918.9 Other and unspecified superficial injuries of eye
921.3 Contusion of eyeball

Applicable HCPCS Level II Codes

A4305 Disposable drug delivery system, flow rate of 50 ml or greater per hour
A4306 Disposable drug delivery system, flow rate of 5 ml or less per hour
A4550 Surgical tray

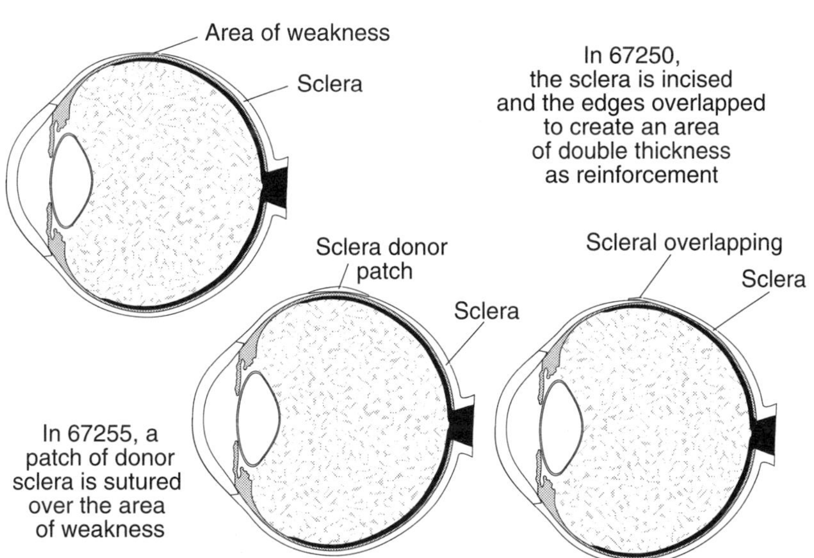

Appendix A Radiology Codes

The codes listed here represent radiology procedures associated with the eye. The CPT code and description are followed by a common language explanation describing the procedure step-by-step in simple terms. The explanation also includes references to related codes in other sections of the book and suggestions on how to avoid common billing errors.

Remember that all radiology codes have a technical and professional component. When physicians do not own their own radiology equipment and thus send their patients to outside testing facilities, they should append modifier -26 to the radiology procedural code to indicate they performed only the professional component.

70030 Radiological examination, eye, for detection of foreign body

The eye is x-rayed for accurate localization of foreign participles lodged within the orbit or eye. There are numerous precision localization techniques devised specifically for this purpose. Each of the numerous methods requires the use of specially designed accessory devices.

70480 Computerized axial tomography, orbit, sella, or posterior fossa or outer middle or inner ear; without contrast material

CT of the orbit allows visualization of abnormalities not readily seen on standard radiographs. Multiple x-rays pass through the orbital area and are measured while detectors record differences in tissue attenuation. The procedure is used to evaluate disease of the orbit and eye; especially lesions.

76511 Ophthalmic ultrasound echography, diagnostic; A-scan only, with amplitude quantification

Ophthalmic ultrasound involves the transmission of high frequency sound waves through the eye and the measurement of the resulting echoes from the ocular structures. An A-scan converts the resulting echoes into waveforms that give a one-dimensional picture. The A-scan is of much greater value in measuring the axial length of the eye and characterizing the tissue texture of abnormal lesions. This test is especially helpful in evaluating cataracts and can identify diseases that may be missed by ophthalmoscopy.

76512 Ophthalmic ultrasound echography, diagnostic; contact B-scan (with or without simultaneous A-scan)

Ophthalmic ultrasound involves the transmission of high-frequency sounds waves through the eye and the measurement of the resulting echoes from the ocular structures. Two types of scans are used. An A-scan converts the resulting echoes into waveforms that give a one-dimensional picture. The A-scan is of much greater value in measuring the axial length of the eye and characterizing the tissue texture of abnormal tissue. B-scan is easier to interpret than the A-scan, and therefore, used more frequently. Thus the combination of A-scans and B-scans produces the most useful test results. The test is especially helpful in evaluating cataracts. Other indications involve hemorrhage, corneal scarring, trauma retinal detachment, intraocular tumor, and other vitreoretinal conditions.

76513 Ophthalmic ultrasound echography diagnostic; immersion (water bath) B-scan

This procedure is an alternative method for performing contact B-scan imaging of the globe using a water bath. The indications include hemorrhage, cataract, corneal scarring and trauma. This procedure can also detect retinal detachment, intraocular tumor and other vitriocorneal conditions.

76516 Ophthalmic biometry by ultrasound echography, A-scan

This procedure uses a probe which performs A-scan only, and is used to determine axial length measurements of the eye.

76519 Ophthalmic biometry by ultrasound echography, A-scan; with intraocular lens power calculation

This procedure uses a probe which performs A-scan only, and is used to determine axial length measurements of the eye for the purpose of evaluating intraocular lens placement and power.

76529 Ophthalmic ultrasonic foreign body localization

This procedure is used when either A-scan or B-scan ophthalmic ultrasound is performed for the purpose of localizing a foreign body and in the guidance for its removal.

Appendix B Path/Lab Codes

The codes listed here represent laboratory and pathology tests commonly associated with the eye. The CPT code and description are followed by a common language explanation. This is by no means a complete list of all the tests that could possibly be performed for conditions affecting the eye, but, rather, a list of those tests most often associated with intraocular surgeries.

87070 Culture, bacterial, definitive; any other source

This test is used to evaluate the causative agent in a suspected infection. A sterile, cotton-tipped swab is used to collect a specimen from the eye. The swab is placed in transport medium. Prior antimicrobial therapy may decrease the yield of organism(s) being cultured.

87184 Sensitivity studies, antibiotic; disk method, per plate (12 or less disks)

This test is of use in the determination of the most effective antibiotic(s) in the treatment of infection of the eye, once the causative organism(s) is identified. Colonies of the isolated organism(s) are subjected to small disks infused with various antibiotics and their susceptibility or resistance are evaluated. A sterile, cotton-tipped swab is used to collect specimen from the eye and placed in transport medium. Prior antimicrobial therapy may interfere with testing.

87186 Sensitivity studies, antibiotic; microtiter, minimum inhibitory concentration (MIC), any number of antibiotics

This test is used to evaluate the most effective antibiotic(s) in the treatment of infection of the eye once the causative organism is identified. Colonies of the isolated organism are introduced to a microtiter plate containing various concentrations of known antibiotics to determine their susceptibility or resistance to the antibiotics and which concentration is most effective. A sterile, cotton-tipped swab containing material taken from eye is submitted for testing. Prior antimicrobial therapy may interfere with testing.

87205 Smear, primary source, with interpretation; routine stain for bacteria, fungi or cell types

This test is used as a preliminary step in the evaluation of which culture medium(s) are indicated to isolate and identify infectious organism(s) in the eye. Slide preparations are prepared from a sterile cotton-tipped swab containing suspected material from the eye and stained according to the type of infection suspected. These slides are examined microscopically to identify the general nature of the causative organism(s). Prior antimicrobial therapy may interfere with testing.

88300 Level I — Surgical pathology, gross examination only

This test is used to evaluate pathological abnormalities in a specimen the examining pathologist determines can be accurately diagnosed without microscopic examination. Specimen tissue obtained during a surgical procedure is submitted for testing. Visual examination by the pathologist is all that is required.

88304 Level III — Surgical pathology, gross and microscopic examination

This test is used to evaluate pathological abnormalities of the conjunctiva, a pterygium, or the cornea. The surgical specimen is submitted for testing. The pathologist performs visual and microscopic examination of the specimen.

88305 Level IV — Surgical pathology, gross and microscopic examination

This test is used to evaluate pathological abnormalities of tissue removed from the eye. Surgical tissue is submitted for testing by gross macroscopic (visual) inspection. This tissue is also microscopically examined by the pathologist.

88307 Level V — Surgical pathology, gross and microscopic examination

This test is used to evaluate pathological abnormalities of an enucleated eye. Suspect tissue obtained during the surgical procedure is submitted for testing for gross macroscopic (visual) inspection. The tissue is also microscopically examined by the pathologist.

88346 Immunofluorescent study, each antibody; direct method

This test is of value in the detection of antibodies to a specific bacterial organism. A sterile, cotton-tipped swab containing suspected infectious material is submitted for testing. Testing is performed by the application of a known antibody to the suspected material and subjected to fluorescent microscopic examination. Prior antimicrobial therapy may interfere with testing.

88347 Immunofluorescent study, each antibody; indirect method

This test is of value in the detection of antibodies to a specific bacterial organism. A sterile, cotton-tipped swab containing suspected material for the eye is submitted for testing. Testing is performed by the application of a known tagged antibody to the suspected material and subjected to florescent microscopic examination. Prior antimicrobial therapy may interfere with testing.

Appendix C HCPCS Codes

HCPCS (pronounced "hick-picks") is an acronym for the HCFA Common Procedure Coding System. HCPCS Level II (national) codes provide a uniform method for reporting medical supplies and equipment as well as select services provided on an outpatient basis.

The following list of codes represents a subset of the entire list of HCPCS Level II codes. The complete list was trimmed down to show only those codes most often associated with the outpatient treatment of the eye.

The first group of codes included in this appendix is the A codes, which are used to report medical and surgical supplies. Next are the J codes assigned to drugs. P codes show pathology and laboratory tests, and K and Q codes represent temporary codes specific to this book. V codes represent vision supplies and services.

When using the J code list, the generic name drug is followed by the brand name, which is enclosed in parentheses. The brand names listed are examples only and may not be inclusive of all products available for that type of drug.

Remember that these codes represent only a partial list of HCPCS Level II codes. They are meant to show the supplies, equipment, and services most commonly associated with the eye. Refer to *HCPCS 1994* for a complete list of Level II codes.

A Codes

A4200 Gauze pads, medicated or nonmedicated, each

A4204 Absorptive dressing (e.g., hydrocolloid), adhesive or nonadhesive

A4205 Nonabsorptive dressing (e.g., hydrogel), adhesive or nonadhesive

A4216 Hemostatic cellulose (e.g., surgical) any size

A4262 Temporary, absorbable lacrimal duct implant, each

A4263 Permanent, long-term, nondissolvable lacrimal duct implant, each

A4305 Disposable drug delivery system, flow rate of 50 ml or greater per hour

A4306 Disposable drug delivery system, flow rate of 5 ml or less per hour

A4550 Surgical tray

A4641 Supply of radiopharmaceutical diagnostic imaging agent

A4644 Supply of low osmolar contrast material (100–199 mg of iodine)

A4645 Supply of low osmolar contrast material (200–299 mg of iodine)

A4646 Supply of low osmolar contrast material (300–399 mg of iodine)

E Codes

E0100 Cane, includes canes of all materials, adjustable or fixed, with tip

J Codes

J0110 Administration of injection, including the cost of drug

J0120 Injection, tetracycline, up to 250 mg (Achromycin)

J0190 Injection, biperiden, 2 mg (Akineton)

J0205 Injection, alglucerase, per 10 units (Ceredase)

J0210 Injection, methyldopate HCl, up to 250 mg (Aldomet)

J0290 Injection, ampicillin, up to 500 mg (Omnipen-N, Polycillin-N, Totacillin-N)

J0300 Injection, amobarbital, up to 125 mg (Amytal)

J0360 Injection, hydralazine HCl, up to 20 mg (Apresoline)

J0380 Injection, metaraminol up to 10 mg (Aramine)

J0390 Injection, chloroquine HCl, up to 50 mg (Aralen)

J0400 Injection, trimethaphan, up to 50 mg (Arfonad)

J0460 Injection, atropine sulfate, up to 0.3 mg

J0520 Injection, bethanechol chloride, up to 5 mg (Urecholine)

J0530 Injection, penicillin G benzathine and penicillin G procaine, up to 600,000 units (Bicillin C-R)

J0540 Injection, penicillin G benzathine and penicilln G procaine, up to 1,200,000 units (Bicillin C-R, Bicillin C-R 900/300)

J0550 Injection, penicillin G benzathine and penicillin G procaine, up to 2,400,000 units (Bicillin C-R)

J0560 Injection, penicillin G benzathine, up to 600,000 units (Bicillin L-A, Permapen)

J0570 Injection, penicillin G benzathine, up to 1,200,000 units (Bicillin L-A, Permapen)

J0580 Injection, penicillin G benzathine, up to 2,400,000 units (Bicillin L-A, Permapen)

J0635 Injection, calcitriol, 1 mcg ampule (Calcijex)

J0670 Injection, Mepivacaine (Carbocaine, Carbocaine with Neo-cobefrin, Polocaine, Isocaine HCl)

J0680 Injection, deslanoside, up to 0.4 mg (Cedilanid-D)

J0690 Injection, cefazolin sodium, up to 500 mg (Ancef, Kefzol, Zolicef)

J0745 Injection, codeine phosphate

J0780 Injection, prochlorperazine, up to 10 mg (Compazine, Cotranzine)

J0895 Injection, deferoxamine mesylate, 500 mg per 5 cc (Desferal Mesylate)

J1205 Injection, chlorothiazide sodium (Diuril Sodium)

J1212 Injection, DMSO, dimethyl sulfoxide

J1330 Injection, ergonovine maleate, up to 0.2 mg

J1340 Injection, aqueous or saline placebo

J1350 Injection, erythromycin-IM, up to 100 mg

J1360 Injection, erthromycin IV, up to 500 mg (Eerythromycin Lactobionate, Erythrocin Lactobionate-IV, Ilotycin Gluceptate)

J1580 Injection, garamycin, gentamicin, up to 80 mg (Gentamicin Sulfate, Jenamicin)

J1640 Injection, heparin sodium, 30 ml (Heparin Lock Flush, Hep-Lock)

J1730 Injection, diazoxide, up to 300 mg (Hyperstat IV)

J1890 Injection, cephalothin sSodium, up to 1 g (Keflin)

J1930 Injection, propiomazine, up to 20 mg (Largon)

J2000 Injection, lidocaine HCl, 50 cc (Xylocaine HCl, Lidoject-1, Lidoject-2, Dilocaine, Caine-1, Caine-2, Nervocaine 1% or ,2%, Nulicaine)

J2010 Injection, lincomycin HCl, up to 300 mg (Lincocin)

J2100 Injection, luminal sodium, up to 120 mg

J2175 Injection, meperidine (Demerol HCl)

J2270 Injection, morphine sulfate, up to 10 mg

J2275 Injection, morphine sulfate (preservative-free sterile solution), per 10 mg (Astramorph PF, Duramorph)

J2400 Injection, chloroprocaine HCl (Nesacaine, Nesacaine-MPF)

J2480 Injection, hydrochlorides of opium alkaloids, up to 20 mg

J2510 Injection, penicillin G procaine, aqueous, up to 600,000 units (Wycillin, Duracillin A.S., Pfizerpen A.S., Crysticillin 300 A.S.)

J2515 Injection, pentobarbital sodium (Nembutal Sodium Solution)

J2520 Injection, thiopental sodium (Pentothal)

J2540 Injection, penicillin G potassium, up to 600,000 units (Pfizerpen)

J2560 Injection, phenobarbital sodium, up to 120 mg

J2860 Injection, secobarbital sodium, up to 250 mg (Seconal)

J3000 Injection, streptomycin, up to 1 g (Streptomycin Sulfate)

J3260 Injection, tobramycin dulfate, up to 80 mg (Nebcin)

J3360 Injection, diazepam, up to 5 mg (Valium, Zetran)

J3364 Injection, urokinase, 5000 IU vial (Abbokinase Open-Cath)

J3365 Injection, IV, urokinase, 250,000 IU vial (Abbokinase)

J3370 Injection, vancomycin HCl, up to 500 mg (Vancocin, Vancoled)

J3420 Injection, vitamin B-12 cyanocobalamin, up to 1000 mcg (Sytobex, Redisol, Rubramin PC, Betalin 12, Berubigen, Cobex)

J3430 Injection, vitamin K, phytonadione, Menadione, menadiol sodium diphosphate (Aqua Mephyton, Konakion, Synkavite)

J3520 Endrate ethylenediamine-tetra-acetic acid (EDTA) (Endrate, Chealamide, Disotate, Edetate Disodium)

J7030 Infusion, normal saline solution, 1000 cc

J7040 Infusion, normal saline solution, sterile (500 ml = 1 unit)

J7042 5 percent dextrose/normal saline (500 ml = 1 unit)

J7050 Infusion, normal saline solution, 250 cc

J7060 5 percent dextrose/water (500 ml = 1 unit) (D-5-W)

J7140 Prescription drug, oral, dispensed in physician's office

J7150 Prescription drug, oral chemotherapy for malignant disease

J9020 Asparaginase, 10,000 units (Elspar)

J9070 Cyclophosphamide, 100 mg (Cytoxan, Neosar)

J9100 Cytarabine, 100 mg (Cytosar-U)

J9240 Medroxyprogesterone acetate, 100 mg (Depo-Provera)

J9270 Plicamycin, 2500 mcg (Mithracin)

J9280 Mitomycin, 5 mg (Mutamycin)

J9293 Mitoxantrone HCle, 20 mg (Novantrone)

J9999 Not otherwise classified, anti-neoplastic drugs

L Codes

L8610 Ocular prosthesis

L8611 Orbital prosthesis

L8612 Aqueous shunt

Q Code

Q0111 Wet mounts, including preparations of vaginal, cervical or skin specimens

V Codes

V2020 Frames, purchases

V2025 Deluxe frame

V2100 Sphere, single vision, plano to plus or minus 4.00, per lens

V2101 Sphere, single vision, plus or minus 4.12 to plus or minus 7.00d,

V2102 Sphere, single vision, plus or minus 7.12 to plus or minus 20.00d,

V2103 Spherocylinder, single vision, plano to plus or minus 4.00d, sphere, 0.12 to 2.00d cylinder, per lens

V2104 Spherocylinder, single vision, plano to plus or minus 4.00d sphere, 2.12 to 4.00d cylinder, per lens

V2105 Spherocylinder, single vision, plano to plus or minus 4.00d sphere, 4.25 to 6.00d cylinder, per lens

V2106 Spherocylinder, single vision, plano to plus or minus 4.00d sphere, over 6.00d cylinder, per lens

V2107 Spherocylinder, single vision, plus or minus 4.25 to plus or minus 7.00 sphere, 0.12 to 2.00d cylinder, per lens

V2108 Spherocylinder, single vision, plus or minus 4.25d to plus or minus 7.00d sphere, 2.12 to 4.00d cylinder, per lens

V2109 Spherocylinder, single vision, plus or minus 4.25 to plus or minus 7.00d sphere, 4.25 to 6.00d cylinder, per lens

V2110 Spherocylinder, single vision, plus or minus 4.25 to 7.00d sphere, over 6.00d cylinder, per lens

V2111 Spherocylinder, single vision, plus or minus 7.25 to plus or minus 12.00d sphere, 0.25 to 2.25d cylinder, per lens

V2112 Spherocylinder, single vision, plus or minus 7.25 to plus or minus 12.00d sphere, 2.25d to 4.00d cylinder, per lens

V2113 Spherocylinder, single vision, plus or minus 7.25 to plus or minus 12.00d sphere, 4.25 to 6.00d cylinder, per lens

V2114 Spherocylinder, single vision sphere over plus or minus 12.00d, per lens

V2115 Lenticular (myodisc), per lens, single vision

V2116 Lenticular lens, nonaspheric, per lens, single vision

V2117 Lenticular, aspheric, per lens, single vision

V2118 Aniseikonic lens, single vision

V2199 Not otherwise classified, single vision lens

V2200 Sphere, bifocal, plano to plus or minus 4.00d, per lens

V2201 Sphere, bifocal, plus or minus 4.12 to plus or minus 7.00d, per lens

V2202 Sphere, bifocal, plus or minus 7.12 to plus or minus 20.00d, per lens

V2203 Spherocylinder, bifocal, plano to plus or minus 4.00d sphere, 0.12 to 2.00d cylinder, per lens

V2204 Spherocylinder, bifocal, plano to plus or minus 4.00d sphere, 2.12 to 4.00d cylinder, per lens

V2205 Spherocylinder, bifocal, plano to plus or minus 4.00d sphere, 4.25 to 6.00d cylinder, per lens

V2206 Spherocylinder, bifocal, plano to plus or minus 4.00d sphere, over 6.00d cylinder, per lens

V2207 Spherocylinder, bifocal, plus or minus 4.25 to plus or minus 7.00d sphere, 0.12 to 2.00d cylinder, per lens

V2208 Spherocylinder, bifocal, plus or minus 4.25 to plus or minus 7.00d sphere, 2.12 to 4.00d cylinder, per lens

V2209 Spherocylinder, bifocal, plus or minus 4.25 to plus or minus 7.00d sphere, 4.25 to 6.00d cylinder, per lens

V2210 Spherocylinder, bifocal, plus or minus 4.25 to plus or minus 7.00d sphere, over 6.00d cylinder, per lens

V2211 Spherocylinder, bifocal, plus or minus 7.25 to plus or minus 12.00d sphere, 0.25 to 2.25d cylinder, per lens

V2212 Spherocylinder, bifocal, plus or minus 7.25 to plus or minus 12.00d sphere, 2.25 to 4.00d cylinder, per lens

V2213 Spherocylinder, bifocal, plus or minus 7.25 to plus or minus 12.00d sphere, 4.25 to 6.00d cylinder, per lens

V2214 Spherocylinder, bifocal, sphere over plus or minus 12.00d, per lens

V2215 Lenticular (myodisc), per lens, bifocal

V2216 Lenticular, nonaspheric, per lens, bifocal

V2217 Lenticular, aspheric lens, bifocal

V2218 Aniseikonic, per lens, bifocal

V2219 Bifocal seg width over 28mm

V2220 Bifocal add over 3.25d

V2299 Specialty bifocal (by report)

V2300 Sphere, trifocal, plano to plus or minus 4.00d, per lens

V2301 Sphere, trifocal, plus or minus 4.12 to plus or minus 7.00d per lens

V2302 Sphere, trifocal, plus or minus 7.12 to plus or minus 20.00, per lens

V2303 Spherocylinder, trifocal, plano to plus or minus 4.00d sphere, 0.12 to 2.00d cylinder, per lens

V2304 Spherocylinder, trifocal, plano to plus or minus 4.00d sphere, 2.25 to 4.00d cylinder, per lens

V2305 Spherocylinder, trifocal, plano to plus or minus 4.00d sphere, 4.25 to 6.00 cylinder, per lens

V2306 Spherocylinder, trifocal, plano to plus or minus 4.00d sphere, over 6.00d cylinder, per lens

V2307 Spherocylinder, trifocal, plus or minus 4.25 to plus or minus 7.00d sphere, 0.12 to 2.00d cylinder, per lens

V2308 Spherocylinder, trifocal, plus or minus 4.25 to plus or minus 7.00d sphere, 2.12 to 4.00d cylinder, per lens

V2309 Spherocylinder, trifocal, plus or minus 4.25 to plus or minus 7.00d sphere, 4.25 to 6.00d cylinder, per lens

V2310 Spherocylinder, trifocal, plus or minus 4.25 to plus or minus 7.00d sphere, over 6.00d cylinder, per lens

V2311 Spherocylinder, trifocal, plus or minus 7.25 to plus or minus 12.00d sphere, 0.25 to 2.25d cylinder, per lens

V2312 Spherocylinder, trifocal, plus or minus 7.25 to plus or minus 12.00d sphere, 2.25 to 4.00d cylinder, per lens

V2313 Spherocylinder, trifocal, plus or minus 7.25 to plus or minus 12.00d sphere, 4.25 to 6.00d cylinder, per lens

V2314 Spherocylinder, trifocal, sphere over plus or minus 12.00d, per lens

V2315 Lenticular (myodisc), per lens, trifocal

V2316 Lenticular nonaspheric, per lens, trifocal

V2317 Lenticular, aspheric lens, trifocal

V2318 Aniseikonic lens, trifocal

V2319 Trifocal seg width over 28 mm

V2320 Trifocal add over 3.25d

V2399 Specialty trifocal (by report)

V2410 Variable asphericity lens, single vision, full field, glass/plastic, per lens

V2430 Variable asphericity lens, bifocal, full field, glass/plastic, per lens

V2499 Variable sphericity lens, other type

V2500 Contact lens, PMMA, spherical, per lens

V2501 Contact lens, PMMA, toric or prism ballast, per lens

V2502 Contact lens, PMMA, bifocal, per lens

V2503 Contact lens, PMMA, color vision deficiency, per lens

V2510 Contact lens, gas permeable, spherical, per lens

V2511 Contact lens, gas permeable, toric, prism ballast, per lens

V2512 Contact lens, gas permeable, bifocal, per lens

V2513 Contact lens, gas permeable, extended wear, per lens

V2520 Contact lens, hydrophilic, spherical, per lens

V2521 Contact lens, hydrophilic, toric, or prism ballast, per lens

V2522 Contact lens, hydrophilic, bifocal, per lens

V2523 Contact lens, hydrophilic, extended wear, per lens

V2530 Contact lens, scleral, per lens (for contact lens modification

V2599 Contact lens, other type

V2600 Hand held low vision aids and other nonspectacle mounted

V2610 Single lens spectacle mounted low vision aids

V2615 Telescopic and other compound lens system, including distance vision telescopic, near vision telescopes and compound microscopic lens system

V2623 Prosthetic eye, plastic, custom

V2624 Polishing/resurfacing of ocular prosthesis

V2625 Enlargement of ocular prosthesis

V2626 Reduction of ocular prosthesis

V2627 Scleral cover shell

V2628 Fabrication and fitting of ocular conformer

V2629 Prosthetic eye, other type

V2630 Anterior chamber intraocular lens

V2631 Iris supported intraocular lens

V2632 Posterior chamber intraocular lens

V2700 Balance lens, per lens

V2710 Slab off prism, glass or plastic, per lens

V2715 Prism, per lens

V2718 Press-on lens, Fresnell prism, per lens

V2730 Special base curve, glass or plastic, per lens

V2740 Tint, plastic, rose 1 or 2, per lens

V2741 Tint, plastic, other than rose 1 or 2, per lens

V2742 Tint, glass, rose 1 or 2, per lens

V2743 Tint, glass, other than rose 1 or 2, per lens

V2744 Tint, photochromatic, per lens

V2750 Antireflective coating, per lens

V2755 U-V lens, per lens

V2760 Scratch resistant coating, per lens

V2770 Occluder lens, per lens

V2780 Oversize lens, per lens

V2785 Processing, preserving and transporting corneal tissue

V2799 Vision service, miscellaneous

Index